I0844294

The Importance of Caregiving For Beginners

By

Tina Cheree Watts

The Importance of Caregiving: Nurturing the Bedrock of Society

Caregiving, often seen as an act of selflessness, involves providing assistance, care, and support to individuals who are unable to fully care for themselves. While caregiving is commonly associated with the elderly or the sick, its significance extends beyond that scope. In fact, caregiving is an essential aspect of society, playing a crucial role in nurturing the well-being and development of individuals across different stages of life. This chapter delves into the importance of caregiving, highlighting its impact on individuals, families, communities, and society as a whole.

Supporting Life's Most Vulnerable:

At its core, caregiving involves ensuring the well-being of those who need it most. Children, the elderly, individuals with disabilities, or those battling chronic illnesses all rely on the unwavering support of caregivers to maintain their dignity and quality of life. Caregivers provide essential assistance with daily tasks, medication management, emotional support, and companionship. By tending to these needs, caregivers allow individuals in vulnerable positions to continue living with respect, comfort, and a sense of independence.

Preserving Family Cohesion:

Caregiving often occurs within the context of the family unit. It is the glue that holds families together, particularly during challenging times. Families that engage in caregiving experience an enhanced sense of unity and togetherness. Taking care of one another fosters stronger emotional bonds, promotes a culture of empathy, nurtures selflessness, and instills values of compassion and altruism in younger generations. Caregiving becomes an opportunity for family members to learn patience, resilience, and a greater understanding of one another's needs.

The Importance of Caregiving for Beginners

Chapter 1: Understanding Caregiving

Introduction to caregiving and its importance. Types of caregivers and their roles, challenges and rewards of being a caregiver.

Chapter 2: Assessing Caregiving Readiness

Self-assessment for potential caregivers. Identifying personal strengths and limitations. Preparing emotionally and mentally for the caregiving journey.

Chapter 3: Creating a Care Plan.

Assessing the care recipient's needs. Building a personalized care plan. Understanding medical and non-medical requirements.

Chapter 4: Navigating Legal and Financial Matters

Legal considerations for caregivers and care recipients. Financial planning and accessing resources. Understanding insurance and benefits.

Chapter 5: Providing Emotional Support

Understanding the emotional needs of care recipients. Managing caregiver stress and burnout. Building a support network.

Chapter 6: Daily Caregiving Skills

Basics of personal care assistance. Administering medications and medical tasks.Safety measures and fall prevention.

Chapter 7: Dealing with Common Health Issues.

Recognizing signs of common health conditions. Managing chronic illnesses and disabilities. Communicating with healthcare professionals effectively.

Chapter 8: Caring for Dementia and Alzheimer's Patients

Understanding dementia and its stages. Strategies for communication and engagement. Creating a dementia-friendly environment.

Chapter 9: Respite Care and Self-Care

Importance of respite care for caregivers. Exploring respite care options. Self-care practices and coping strategies.

Chapter 10: Transitioning and Grief

Preparing for end-of-life decisions. Coping with grief and loss. Celebrating the caregiving journey.

Economic Impact:

Besides its pivotal role within the family, caregiving has a profound economic impact. Family members who assume caregiving roles often save society incredible sums of money that would otherwise be spent on professional care services. According to the AARP, family caregivers provide an estimated $470 billion worth of unpaid care annually in the United States alone. This immense contribution significantly relieves the burden on healthcare and social welfare systems, allowing resources to be allocated where they are most needed. By lessening the demand on public services, caregiving enables effective resource management and helps maintain a sustainable and balanced society.

Community Building:

Caregiving extends its reach beyond the family unit, spilling into the wider community. Neighbors, friends, or volunteers who offer their time and support to those in need play a crucial role in strengthening community ties. Communities that embrace caregiving foster an atmosphere of reciprocity, social cohesion, and collective responsibility. Supporting individuals in need not only addresses their immediate challenges but also creates a domino effect, encouraging others to contribute to their community positively. Communities that value caregiving and provide an infrastructure to support caregivers create an environment that nourishes trust, kindness, and solidarity.

Promoting Mental and Emotional Well-being:

Caregiving is a challenging endeavor that often requires substantial physical, mental, and emotional efforts. It demands resilience, patience, adaptability, and sacrifice from those who take on the role of caregivers. However, it is through this journey that caregivers often discover their inner strength and develop a profound sense of fulfillment. The act of caring for another human being promotes personal growth, empathy, and gratitude. Caregivers gain a deeper understanding of their own values, priorities, and purpose in life.

Caregiving is an invaluable cornerstone of society. It encompasses both a nurturing role and a profound responsibility. Beyond the immediate influence on individuals and families, caregiving has far-reaching effects, promoting economic stability, community cohesion, and personal growth. As societies continue to evolve and face new challenges, recognizing and supporting caregiving becomes crucial. By providing the necessary resources, recognition, and support to caregivers, societies can create a future where individuals thrive, communities flourish, and the very fabric of society remains tightly woven by the bonds of compassion.

Types of Caregivers and Their Roles: Allies in Caring

Caregiving is a multifaceted role that encompasses a wide range of responsibilities and specialized skills. Different care needs require various types of caregivers, each with their own unique expertise and focus. Understanding the different types of caregivers and their roles is instrumental in providing appropriate and effective care for individuals in diverse situations. This chapter explores the various types of caregivers, from informal family caregivers to professional healthcare providers, highlighting the significance of their roles in supporting those in need.

1. Informal Family Caregivers:

Informal family caregivers are often the backbone of the care system, fulfilling their roles out of love, duty, and a sense of responsibility. They are usually family members, such as spouses, children, siblings, or close relatives, who assume caregiving responsibilities without formal training or compensation. Their commitment and dedication are unparalleled, as they provide emotional support, perform daily tasks, and coordinate medical care. Informal family caregivers fill vital roles in the lives of their loved ones, offering assistance with personal care, transportation, household tasks, medication management, and companionship.

2. Professional Healthcare Providers:

a) Home Health Aides and Personal Care Assistants:

Home health aides and personal care assistants are trained professionals who provide essential care in individuals' homes. They assist with bathing, dressing, toileting, medication administration, and daily living activities. Their focus is on maintaining the comfort and overall well-being of individuals while adhering to professional standards and regulations.

b) Nurses:

Registered Nurses (RNs) and Licensed Practical Nurses (LPNs) play critical roles in caregiving, providing medical care, administering medications, monitoring vital signs, and coordinating treatments. Nurses are well-versed in assessing patient needs, identifying potential health risks, and implementing appropriate interventions. Their expertise extends beyond physical care, as they also provide emotional support to individuals and their families.

c) Certified Nursing Assistants (CNAs):

Certified Nursing Assistants work under the supervision of nurses and provide direct patient care, including assistance with daily activities, mobility support, and personal hygiene. CNAs play essential roles in healthcare settings, ensuring individuals' comfort, safety, and basic needs are met.

d) Physical Therapists, Occupational Therapists, and Speech-Language Pathologists:

These specialized healthcare professionals focus on rehabilitation and improving individuals' physical and cognitive abilities. Physical therapists help restore and enhance mobility, occupational therapists assist individuals in regaining independence in daily tasks, and speech-language pathologists work with those facing communication or swallowing difficulties. Their expertise is vital in the recovery and well-being of individuals with injuries, disabilities, or other medical conditions.

3. Respite Care Providers:

Respite care providers offer temporary relief and support to primary caregivers, allowing them to take breaks, attend to personal needs, or simply recharge. This type of caregiving is usually provided by trained professionals or volunteers. Respite care not only helps prevent caregiver burnout but also ensures the continuity of quality care for individuals who require constant support.

4. Hospice Care Teams:

Hospice care teams consist of physicians, nurses, social workers, spiritual counselors, and volunteers who work together to provide comfort and support to individuals with terminal illnesses and their families. These teams focus on pain and symptom management, emotional and spiritual guidance, and enhancing individuals' quality of life during their final stages. Hospice care emphasizes compassion, dignity, and supporting individuals to live their remaining days with comfort and grace.

Caregiving is a complex and diverse field, encompassing a range of roles and expertise. From informal family caregivers invested in love and dedication to professional healthcare providers trained in specialized forms of care, each type of caregiver plays a crucial role in supporting individuals in need. Recognizing and appreciating the contributions of different caregivers is essential in creating a comprehensive and effective care system. By working together in harmony, caregivers of all types become allies, providing holistic, compassionate care to those who rely on their expertise and support.

The Challenges of Being a Caregiver

Being a caregiver is an honorable and selfless role that involves providing support, assistance, and care to individuals who are unable to fully care for themselves. While the act of caregiving is often associated with compassion and love, it is not without its challenges. Caregivers face numerous obstacles on their caregiving journey, which can impact their physical, emotional, and mental well-being. This chapter explores the challenges that caregivers commonly encounter and emphasizes the need for support systems and resources to address these difficulties.

1. Physical Demands:

Caregiving often involves physical tasks such as lifting, bathing, toileting, and assisting with mobility. These activities can be physically demanding, especially when caring for individuals with limited mobility or those who require constant attention. Caregivers may experience physical strain, fatigue, and even the risk of injury. The demanding nature of caregiving can take a toll on the caregiver's own health and well-being, making it essential for caregivers to prioritize self-care and seek assistance when needed.

2. Emotional and Mental Strain:

Witnessing a loved one's struggles, deterioration of health, or decline in cognitive abilities can cause immense emotional and mental strain for caregivers. They may experience feelings of sadness, grief, frustration, guilt, and helplessness. The emotional rollercoaster of caregiving, coupled with the pressure to provide the best possible care, can lead to caregiver burnout, anxiety, depression, and feelings of isolation. It is essential that caregivers have access to emotional support, counseling, or a support network to help them navigate the complex emotions they may experience.

3. Time and Financial Constraints:

Caregiving is a time-intensive responsibility, often requiring round-the-clock care and attention. Balancing caregiving responsibilities with other aspects of life, such as work, personal relationships, and self-care, can be incredibly challenging. Many caregivers find themselves juggling multiple roles, which can lead to feelings of overwhelm and exhaustion. Moreover, caregiving often incurs significant financial costs, including medical expenses, specialized equipment, and home modifications. Financial strain can further add to the challenges that caregivers face, necessitating access to resources and financial assistance.

4. Lack of Support and Recognition:

Caregivers often face a lack of understanding and recognition for the vital role they play in society. Many caregivers feel isolated and unsupported, which can exacerbate the burden they carry. Frustration may arise from a lack of external empathy, as others may not fully comprehend the physical, emotional, and mental toll that caregiving entails. Building a support network, connecting with other caregivers, and advocating for increased awareness and recognition can help alleviate this challenge.

5. Role Strain and Identity Shift:

Caregiving often necessitates significant lifestyle changes and shifts in personal identity. Caregivers may find it challenging to navigate their own needs, aspirations, and personal relationships while dedicating themselves to the care of another. Struggling to maintain a sense of self and a balance between caregiving responsibilities and personal fulfillment can lead to feelings of loss, identity crisis, and strained relationships. Respite care, professional counseling, and self-reflection can support caregivers in finding equilibrium between their caregiver role and personal aspirations.

Being a caregiver is a noble yet demanding role. Caregivers face numerous challenges, including the physical demands of caregiving, emotional and mental strain, time and financial constraints, lack of support, and identity shifts. Recognizing and addressing these challenges is essential to support caregivers in their selfless endeavors. Society must provide caregiver support programs, access to respite care, and avenues for emotional and financial assistance. By understanding and meeting the needs of caregivers, we can contribute to their overall well-being and ensure the sustainability of caregiving efforts. Ultimately, supporting caregivers benefits not only the individuals they care for but also society as a whole.

The Rewards of Being a Caregiver

Caregiving, while undeniably challenging, also offers numerous rewards and fulfilling experiences. It is a role that allows individuals to make a positive difference in the lives of others, promoting their well-being, independence, and quality of life. This chapter explores the rewards that come with being a caregiver and highlights the intrinsic value and personal growth that can be achieved through caregiving.

1. Making a Significant Impact:

One of the most gratifying aspects of being a caregiver is the opportunity to positively impact someone's life. Caregiving allows individuals to provide essential support, comfort, and care to those in need. Witnessing the improvement in an individual's health, well-being, and overall outlook on life can be incredibly rewarding. Having the ability to make even a small difference in someone's daily life or journey toward recovery can be immensely fulfilling.

2. Building Deep Connections:

Caregiving fosters profound connections between the caregiver and the individual receiving care. Spending quality time together, engaging in meaningful conversations, sharing experiences, and providing emotional support can create bonds that are both powerful and lasting. These connections often nurture a sense of purpose, belonging, and joy in the lives of both the caregiver and the care recipient.

3. Learning and Personal Growth:

Caregiving offers countless opportunities for personal growth and learning. Caregivers develop resilience, patience, empathy, and adaptability through the challenges they face. They become adept problem-solvers, equipped with the ability to think on their feet and handle unexpected situations. Caregivers also learn to prioritize self-care and their own well-being while simultaneously caring for others. This personal growth translates into various aspects of life, enhancing their relationships, professional skills, and overall sense of accomplishment.

4. Gaining a Deeper Appreciation for Life:

Caregiving can provide a fresh perspective on life and a heightened appreciation for its precious moments. Seeing the courage and strength of individuals facing adversity can inspire caregivers to embrace gratitude, mindfulness, and a renewed zest for life. Caregivers often become more attuned to the values that truly matter, prioritizing love, compassion, and the importance of human connection.

5. An Opportunity for Self-Discovery:

Caregiving also presents caregivers with the chance to discover their true strengths, talents, and passions. It provides an avenue for individuals to explore their innate capacity for caregiving, empathy, and nurturing. Many caregivers find a sense of purpose and fulfillment in their role, discovering their life's calling and finding profound meaning in their everyday actions.

While being a caregiver undoubtedly presents its share of challenges, it also offers immense rewards and personal growth. The ability to positively impact someone's life, build deep connections, learn and grow, gain a deeper appreciation for life, and engage in self-discovery makes the caregiving journey invaluable. Society must recognize and celebrate the rewards of caregiving, providing support systems and resources that enable caregivers to fulfill their responsibilities effectively. By acknowledging and valuing caregivers, we can foster a culture of appreciation and support, ensuring that the rewards of caregiving continue to enrich the lives of both caregivers and those under their care.

Chapter 2

Assessing Caregiving Readiness

Before embarking on the journey of caregiving, it is crucial to assess one's readiness for this significant responsibility. Assessing caregiving readiness helps individuals determine if they possess the emotional, practical, and financial capabilities required to provide effective care. This chapter explores various factors to consider when assessing caregiving readiness.

1. Emotional Readiness:

Emotional readiness is the foundation upon which effective caregiving is built. To assess emotional readiness, one must consider their ability to cope with stress, uncertainty, and the emotional impact of providing care. Asking oneself the following questions can aid in this assessment:

- Am I able to handle emotional and physical challenges that may arise during caregiving?

- How well do I manage stress, frustration, and potential feelings of isolation?

- Can I remain empathetic, patient, and supportive when dealing with the care recipient's emotions and needs?

- Am I willing to seek emotional support when needed to maintain my own well-being?

2. Practical Readiness:

Practical readiness encompasses the knowledge, skills, and resources required to provide adequate care. Assessing practical readiness involves considering the following factors:

- Do I possess the necessary knowledge about the care recipient's condition, medical needs, and any associated tasks, such as administering medication or performing medical procedures?

- Am I prepared to learn and acquire new skills, such as using assistive devices or managing medical equipment?

- Do I have access to relevant resources, such as medical supplies, assistive devices, or home modifications?

- Can I effectively communicate and collaborate with healthcare professionals and support networks?

3. Financial Readiness:

Assessing financial readiness involves considering the financial implications of caregiving and evaluating one's ability to provide the necessary support without compromising their own financial stability. Some questions for consideration include:

- Have I considered the potential costs associated with caregiving, such as medical expenses, modifications to the living environment, or transportation expenses?

- Can I manage my own financial obligations while also covering the additional expenses that may arise from caregiving?

- Are there any available financial assistance programs or resources that can help alleviate the financial burden of caregiving?

4. Assessing Potential Challenges:

It is crucial to anticipate and prepare for potential challenges that may arise during caregiving. Some common challenges include caregiver burnout, strain on personal relationships, and managing conflicts within the caregiving dynamic. Assessing potential challenges can involve reflecting on the following questions:

- Am I aware of the potential physical, emotional, and social challenges associated with caregiving?

- Can I identify support systems and resources that can help alleviate these challenges?

- How will I manage and prioritize my own self-care while providing care to the care recipient?

Assessing caregiving readiness is an essential step in becoming a competent and effective caregiver. Emotional, practical, and financial readiness, as well as an awareness of potential challenges, contribute to an individual's ability to provide optimal care. By honestly evaluating their readiness, individuals can make informed decisions and take necessary steps to ensure the well-being of both themselves and the care recipient throughout the caregiving journey.

Caregiving readiness is a crucial aspect of ensuring the well-being and quality of life for those in need. It involves being adequately prepared, both emotionally and practically, to take on the responsibilities and challenges associated with caring for someone who requires assistance. Caregiving can encompass a wide range of tasks, from providing physical care to addressing emotional needs, and it often requires significant commitment, time, and effort. Therefore, a strong sense of readiness is essential to ensure that the caregiver can provide the best possible support.

Emotional readiness is one of the first considerations when it comes to caregiving. It is important to assess one's own emotional capacity and stability before taking on the responsibility of caring for another individual. Providing care can be emotionally demanding, as it often involves witnessing the struggles and challenges faced by the person being cared for. This can include physical pain, cognitive decline, or emotional distress. Caregivers must be prepared to handle these emotions and provide support to the best of their abilities while still maintaining their own well-being.

Practical readiness is another crucial aspect of caregiving. This includes being knowledgeable about the specific needs of the person requiring care and having the necessary skills to provide appropriate assistance. For example, if caring for an elderly individual, one must be prepared to assist with activities of daily living, such as bathing, dressing, and medication management. Practical readiness also involves having a basic understanding of medical conditions and being able to communicate effectively with healthcare professionals. Furthermore, caregivers need to ensure they have access to necessary resources, such as medical supplies, assistive devices, or support networks, to ensure they can meet the needs of the care recipient effectively.

Financial readiness is another important consideration when it comes to caregiving. Providing care can often come with financial implications, such as medical expenses, transportation costs, or modifications to the living environment. Caregivers need to assess their financial situation and plan accordingly to ensure they can provide the necessary support without compromising their own financial stability.

In addition to emotional, practical, and financial preparedness, caregivers should also be aware of potential challenges and develop strategies to address them. These challenges can include burnout, feelings of isolation, or conflict within the caregiving relationship. Being aware of potential difficulties allows caregivers to seek support, both professional and personal, to cope with the demands of caregiving. This may include joining support groups, seeking respite care, or accessing counseling services.

Lastly, caregivers must also consider their own personal well-being. It is crucial to maintain one's physical and mental health while providing care for others. This may involve seeking regular medical check-ups, practicing self-care, and setting boundaries to prevent overwhelm or exhaustion. Caregivers who neglect their own well-being may not be able to provide the best quality of care to those they are caring for.

Caregiving readiness is essential for those who take on the responsibility of caring for others. Emotional readiness, practical readiness, financial readiness, and awareness of potential challenges all contribute to creating a solid foundation for successful caregiving. Caregivers who are adequately prepared are more likely to provide the best possible support, leading to improved well-being and quality of life for both the care recipient and the caregiver themselves.

Chapter 3

Creating a Care Plan

Once a caregiver has assessed their readiness and determined that they are prepared to take on the responsibility of caring for someone, the next step is to create a comprehensive care plan. A care plan provides a roadmap for ensuring that all aspects of the care recipient's needs are met effectively and efficiently. This chapter explores the process of creating a care plan and its importance in caregiving.

1. Assessing the Care Recipient's Needs:

The first step in creating a care plan is to conduct a thorough assessment of the care recipient's needs. This involves evaluating their physical, emotional, and cognitive abilities and identifying any specific healthcare requirements. Questions to consider during this assessment include:

- What are the care recipient's daily living needs, such as personal hygiene, dressing, and meal preparation?

- Do they have any medical conditions or disabilities that require specialized care, such as medication administration or physical therapy?

- Are they experiencing cognitive decline or memory loss that may impact their ability to make decisions or perform daily tasks?

- What are their emotional needs and how can they be supported?

2. Setting Goals and Objectives:

Once the care recipient's needs have been identified, the caregiver can set goals and objectives for the care plan. This involves establishing what the caregiver hopes to achieve and outlining specific actions to accomplish these goals. Some examples of goals and objectives may include:

- Improving the care recipient's overall quality of life by providing consistent emotional support.

- Assisting with daily living activities to promote independence and maintain a sense of dignity.

- Managing and monitoring medical conditions to prevent complications and improve overall health.

- Ensuring the care recipient's safety by implementing necessary home modifications and providing supervision.

3. Identifying Resources and Support:

Caregivers must identify the resources and support needed to execute the care plan. This may include:

- Medical professionals: Establishing relationships with healthcare providers, including primary care physicians, specialists, therapists, or nurses, who can offer guidance and support.

- Community resources: Exploring local resources such as senior centers, adult day care programs, and support groups can provide additional assistance and relief for caregivers.

- Financial support: Assessing available financial resources and exploring potential assistance programs, insurance coverage, or government benefits to alleviate the financial burden of caregiving.

4. Implementing the Care Plan:

Once all necessary resources and support systems are in place, the caregiver can begin implementing the care plan. This involves putting the goals and objectives into action, following any medical or therapeutic protocols, and ensuring that all necessary care is provided. It is important to regularly review and update the care plan as the care recipient's needs and circumstances change.

5. Regular Evaluation and Adjustments:

A care plan should be a dynamic document that is regularly evaluated and adjusted as needed. The caregiver should continuously monitor the care recipient's progress and adapt the plan accordingly. Regular communication with healthcare professionals, the care recipient, and their support network is essential to ensure that the care plan remains effective and addresses any new or changing needs.

Creating a care plan is an integral part of caregiving, as it provides structure and guidance to ensure that all aspects of the care recipient's needs are met. By conducting a thorough assessment, setting goals, identifying resources, and regularly evaluating the plan, caregivers can provide the best possible care to enhance the well-being and quality of life for the individual they are caring for.

Caregivers often find themselves navigating complex legal and financial matters while providing care for their loved ones. They may encounter a range of legal concerns, such as understanding and executing power of attorney documents, managing healthcare proxies, or navigating guardianship issues. Additionally, caregivers may need to handle financial matters, including managing the care recipient's expenses, accessing insurance benefits, or applying for government assistance programs. Navigating these legal and financial matters can be daunting, but with the help of legal and financial professionals, caregivers can ensure they are making informed decisions and taking the necessary steps to protect the best interests of their loved ones.

Caregivers Navigating Legal and Financial Matters

Caregiving comes with a host of legal and financial responsibilities that can be overwhelming for caregivers. Navigating these matters is crucial to ensure the well-being and protection of both the caregiver and the care recipient. This chapter explores the key legal and financial considerations caregivers should be aware of and offers guidance on effectively managing these complex aspects of caregiving.

1. Understanding Legal Matters:

a. Power of Attorney: Understanding and executing power of attorney documents is crucial for caregivers. This legal document grants the caregiver the authority to make financial and healthcare decisions on behalf of the care recipient. It is essential to consult with an attorney to ensure the power of attorney is properly drafted and executed.

b. Healthcare Proxies and Advanced Directives: Healthcare proxies and advanced directives allow the care recipient to designate someone to make medical decisions in the event they are unable to do so. Caregivers should ensure these documents are in place and readily accessible when needed.

c. Guardianship: In some cases, caregivers may need to navigate the process of obtaining legal guardianship if the care recipient is unable to make decisions independently. This entails working with an attorney to petition the court and provide evidence that guardianship is necessary.

2. Managing Financial Matters:

a. Budgeting and Expense Management: Caregivers should establish a budget and financial plan to effectively manage the care recipient's expenses and ensure their financial stability. This may involve tracking expenses, seeking professional advice, and exploring resources for financial assistance.

b. Insurance and Benefits: Caregivers should become well-versed in the care recipient's insurance coverage, including health insurance, long-term care insurance, and disability benefits. Understanding the scope of coverage, filing claims, and advocating for appropriate benefits is essential.

c. Government Assistance Programs: Caregivers should explore government assistance programs that can provide financial support for both the care recipient and caregiver. This includes programs such as Medicaid, Medicare, Social Security, and Veterans Benefits. Researching eligibility criteria, application processes, and required documentation is vital to accessing these resources.

3. Legal and Financial Professionals:

Seeking guidance from legal and financial professionals is crucial for caregivers to navigate these complex matters effectively. Engaging lawyers specializing in elder law or estate planning can help ensure legal documents are in order and provide guidance on legal issues that may arise. Additionally, financial advisors or certified public accountants can help with financial planning, tax considerations, and maximizing available resources.

4. Communication and Documentation:

Clear communication and proper documentation are key to resolving legal and financial matters efficiently. Maintaining detailed records of expenses, medical documents, legal documents, and communication with professionals is essential. This information will be invaluable in case of audits, insurance claims, or disputes.

5. Self-Care and Support:

Navigating legal and financial matters can be stressful for caregivers. It is crucial to prioritize self-care and seek emotional support through counseling, support groups, or friends and family. Additionally, considering respite care options to temporarily relieve caregiving responsibilities can alleviate some of the stress associated with these matters.

Caregivers must navigate a range of legal and financial matters to ensure the well-being and protection of the care recipient and themselves. By understanding legal documents, managing financial matters effectively, seeking professional guidance, and prioritizing self-care, caregivers can navigate these challenges with confidence and ensure the best possible outcomes for both the care recipient and themselves.

Legal Considerations for the Caregiver and the Care Recipient

Caring for a loved one involves not only providing physical and emotional support but also navigating various legal considerations. Understanding and addressing these legal matters are essential for both the caregiver and the care recipient. This chapter explores key legal considerations and offers guidance on how to navigate them effectively.

1. Power of Attorney:

A power of attorney (POA) is a legal document that designates an individual to make financial and legal decisions on behalf of the care recipient. Caregivers should ensure that the care recipient has a valid and up-to-date POA in place. It is crucial to consult an attorney specializing in elder law to properly establish, execute, and understand the responsibilities and limitations of this document.

2. Healthcare Decision-Making:

The care recipient's ability to make medical decisions may become limited over time. It is essential to address healthcare decision-making in advance. This can be done through documents such as a healthcare proxy or a living will, which outline the care recipient's wishes and assign a trusted individual to make medical decisions when they are unable to do so. Consulting with an attorney specializing in healthcare directives can guide caregivers through this process.

3. Guardianship:

In some cases, when a care recipient is unable to make decisions independently and there is no valid POA or healthcare directive in place, the caregiver may need to seek guardianship. Guardianship is a legal process that grants the caregiver authority to make decisions on behalf of the care recipient. However, it is a complex process and usually requires involvement with the court system. Consulting with an attorney experienced in guardianship matters is highly recommended.

4. Estate Planning:

Estate planning ensures the care recipient's assets and wishes are protected and carried out accordingly. This may involve creating a will, establishing trusts, designating beneficiaries, or updating existing documents. Caregivers should encourage the care recipient to consult with an estate planning attorney to ensure their assets are distributed as desired and potential tax implications are considered.

5. Elder Abuse and Fraud Protection:

Caregivers should be vigilant about protecting the care recipient from potential elder abuse and fraud. They should familiarize themselves with warning signs, educate the care recipient on common scams, and take necessary precautions to safeguard financial and personal information. Reporting any suspected abuse or fraudulent activities to appropriate authorities is essential.

6. Legal Contracts and Agreements:

Caregivers may need to enter into legal contracts or agreements, such as home care contracts or caregiver employment agreements. These documents outline the terms and conditions of the caregiver's role, responsibilities, and compensation. Seeking legal advice and having these contracts properly drafted can protect both the caregiver's and the care recipient's interests.

7. Legal Assistance and Support:

Caregivers should seek legal assistance when needed, as the intricacies of legal matters can be overwhelming. Engaging an attorney experienced in elder law or estate planning can provide invaluable guidance and ensure legal matters are addressed accurately and ethically.

Legal considerations play a vital role in caregiving and ensuring the rights and well-being of both the caregiver and the care recipient. Understanding and addressing legal matters, such as powers of attorney, healthcare decision-making, guardianship, estate planning, fraud protection, contracts, and legal assistance, are crucial steps in providing comprehensive care. By seeking professional legal advice and engaging in proactive planning, caregivers can navigate these considerations effectively, providing the best possible care for their loved ones.

Caregiver's Financial Planning and Accessing Resources

As a caregiver, your role in supporting a loved one is not only emotionally fulfilling but also entails managing various financial aspects. Caregiving can often create financial strain, both in terms of daily expenses and long-term planning. This chapter aims to guide you through the process of financial planning and accessing relevant resources efficiently. By adopting these proactive steps, you can ensure financial stability while providing the care your loved one deserves.

1. Establishing a Solid Financial Foundation:

Before delving into your loved one's specific needs, ensure your personal finances are on solid footing. Assess your own financial stability by tracking your income, expenses, and debts. Create a budget to identify areas where you can save and cut unnecessary expenses. An emergency fund is crucial to cover unexpected costs that may arise, thereby avoiding financial distress.

2. Assessing Your Loved One's Financial Situation:

To support your loved one effectively, it is essential to understand their financial position. Begin by gathering information on their income, assets, benefits, and expenses. Compile this data into a comprehensive overview that outlines their financial resources. Review existing insurance policies, including health, disability, and long-term care coverage, to determine if additional coverage is necessary.

3. Engaging Professional Assistance:

Financial planning can be complex, especially when combined with caregiving responsibilities. Consider seeking professional advice from financial planners or elder law attorneys specializing in senior care. These experts can provide guidance on long-term financial strategies, government benefits, estate planning, and tax implications.

4. Exploring Government Assistance Programs:

Numerous government programs offer financial assistance to caregivers and their loved ones. Research eligibility requirements and explore programs such as Medicaid, Medicare, Social Security Disability Insurance (SSDI), Supplemental Security Income (SSI), and Veterans Affairs (VA) benefits. These programs can help alleviate the financial burden associated with healthcare and long-term care costs.

5. Understanding Tax Deductions and Credits:

Tax planning is crucial for caregivers, as you may be eligible for deductions and credits. Investigate tax provisions applicable to caregivers, such as the caregiver tax credit and deductions for medical expenses and home modifications. Consult a tax professional or utilize reliable tax software to ensure you maximize your benefits while remaining compliant with tax regulations.

6. Utilizing Community Resources:

Local community organizations and nonprofit agencies often provide resources to support caregivers and their loved ones. These resources may include respite care services, support groups, educational workshops, and financial counseling. Connecting with these organizations can provide valuable guidance and assistance, ultimately reducing financial stress.

7. Exploring Long-Term Care Options:

Research different long-term care options available to your loved one, such as assisted living facilities, in-home care services, or adult day programs. Understand the cost implications associated with each option by gathering estimates and scrutinizing their financial feasibility. To finance long-term care, you can consider long-term care insurance, reverse mortgages, or veterans' benefits.

Caregiving demands substantial time and resources, making financial planning an essential aspect of caregiving responsibilities. Empower yourself with the knowledge necessary to make informed financial decisions. By understanding your own financial situation, exploring government programs, accessing community resources, and seeking expert advice, you can successfully navigate the financial challenges associated with caregiving and ensure the highest level of care for your loved one. Remember, proactive financial planning not only benefits your loved one but also safeguard your financial well-being.

Caregivers Understanding Insurance and Benefits

One of the key aspects of providing effective care as a caregiver is understanding the intricacies of insurance and benefits. Navigating the world of insurance and benefits can be complex, but having a solid understanding of these areas will help you access the resources and support necessary to provide the best care for your loved one. This chapter aims to guide you through the process of understanding insurance and benefits so that you can confidently advocate for your loved one's needs.

1. Health Insurance Coverage:

Understanding your loved one's health insurance coverage is crucial since it plays a pivotal role in managing medical expenses. Review their health insurance policy to understand the extent of coverage, including doctor visits, hospital stays, medications, and specialized treatments. Familiarize yourself with co-pays, deductibles, and out-of-pocket maximums to accurately estimate potential costs.

2. Long-Term Care Insurance:

Long-term care insurance is specifically designed to cover the costs associated with extended care services such as home care, assisted living, or nursing homes. If your loved one has this type of insurance, thoroughly review the policy to understand the covered services, elimination period, benefit limits, and any waiting periods. Determine if the policy requires specific qualifications for reimbursement and, if needed, seek advice from an insurance professional specializing in long-term care.

3. Government Benefits:

There are several government programs that provide benefits to individuals requiring care. Research and understand eligibility requirements for programs such as Medicaid, Medicare, Social Security Disability Insurance (SSDI), and Supplemental Security Income (SSI). Each program has its own set of rules and regulations, so it is crucial to become familiar with these programs to maximize your loved one's benefits.

4. Veterans Benefits:

If your loved one is a veteran, they may be eligible for additional benefits through the Department of Veterans Affairs (VA). Investigate the various VA programs, such as the Aid and Attendance benefit or the Veterans Directed Home and Community-Based Services (VD-HCBS), to gain a comprehensive understanding of the support available. Consult with a VA representative or veterans service organization to assist with the application process.

5. Employer Benefits:

Determine if your loved one has access to any employer-provided benefits that could assist with healthcare costs or caregiving expenses. Review employee benefits such as health insurance, flexible spending accounts (FSAs), health savings accounts (HSAs), or employee assistance programs (EAPs). Speak with the human resources department or benefits manager to obtain complete information and understand how to maximize the available benefits.

6. Coordination of Benefits:

If your loved one has multiple insurance coverages, it is necessary to understand how these policies coordinate with one another. Insurance policies often have specific coordination of benefits rules to determine the primary and secondary payers. This knowledge can help ensure claims are correctly submitted and reduce any potential billing confusion.

7. Utilizing Advocate Services:

If you find the process of understanding insurance and benefits overwhelming, consider engaging the services of professional advocates. Insurance advocates or patient navigators specialize in helping individuals understand and navigate insurance-related matters. These professionals can guide you through the insurance landscape, advocate for claims and reimbursements, and help resolve any disputes or billing issues.

Understanding insurance and benefits is crucial for caregivers to ensure adequate coverage and access to essential resources. Thoroughly reviewing health insurance policies, exploring long-term care insurance options, researching government programs and veterans' benefits, and understanding employer benefits will help you make informed decisions. Coordinating benefits and utilizing advocate services when necessary will further streamline the insurance process. By becoming well-versed in insurance and benefits, you will be better equipped to advocate for your loved one's needs and successfully navigate the complexities of healthcare and caregiving expenses.

Chapter 5

Providing Emotional Support

Providing Emotional Support as a Caregiver

As a caregiver, your role goes beyond providing physical care for your loved one. Emotional support plays a vital role in their well-being and overall quality of life. This chapter aims to guide you on how to provide effective and meaningful emotional support, ensuring your loved one feels understood, validated, and cared for throughout their journey.

1. Active Listening:

One of the most powerful ways to provide emotional support is through active listening. Be fully present when engaging in conversations with your loved one. Give them your undivided attention, maintain eye contact, and listen attentively to their thoughts, concerns, and feelings. Show empathy and validate their emotions, allowing them to express themselves openly without fear of judgment.

2. Encourage Expression:

Create a safe and non-judgmental space for your loved one to express their emotions freely. Encourage them to share their thoughts, fears, and worries openly. Let them know that it is okay to experience a range of emotions and that you are there to support and understand them. Avoid dismissing or minimizing their feelings, as this can invalidate their experiences.

3. Foster a Supportive Environment:

Create an environment that fosters emotional well-being and promotes positivity. Engage in activities that bring joy and uplift spirits. Encourage hobbies, interests, and social interactions that help your loved one maintain a sense of purpose and fulfillment. Surround them with positive influences, such as uplifting music, inspiring books, and supportive friends or family members.

4. Practice Empathy:

Put yourself in your loved one's shoes and try to understand their perspective. Empathy allows you to connect with their emotions and experiences on a deeper level. Validate their feelings by acknowledging their challenges, fears, and frustrations. Offer words of comfort and reassurance, showing understanding and compassion.

5. Encourage Self-Care:

Help your loved one prioritize self-care as a means of managing their emotional well-being. Encourage them to engage in activities that bring them joy and relaxation, such as pursuing hobbies, reading, meditating, or spending time in nature. Remind them of the importance of taking breaks and caring for themselves in order to recharge and maintain emotional resilience.

6. Provide Emotional Validation:

Validate your loved one's emotional experiences by acknowledging their feelings and reinforcing their strengths. Remind them that their emotions are valid and understandable, given the circumstances. Avoid judgment or criticism and instead focus on helping them find healthy ways to cope and process their emotions effectively.

7. Seek Professional Support:

Recognize when your loved one may benefit from additional emotional support beyond what you can provide. Encourage them to seek therapy or counseling services to facilitate a safe and unbiased space for them to address their emotions and mental well-being. Professional support can offer valuable tools and strategies to help them navigate their emotions and overcome challenges.

Providing emotional support is an essential aspect of caregiving, helping your loved one navigate the emotional ups and downs of their journey. By actively listening, encouraging expression, fostering a supportive environment, practicing empathy, promoting self-care, providing emotional validation, and seeking professional support when needed, you create an environment of understanding and compassion. Remember that emotional support is an ongoing process, and being there for your loved one in both the good times and the difficult moments will make a significant difference in their overall well-being.

Understanding the Emotional Needs of Care Recipients

When providing care to a loved one, it is crucial to recognize and understand their emotional needs. These needs can often be overlooked while focusing on physical care. This chapter aims to guide caregivers in understanding the emotional needs of care recipients, ensuring a holistic approach towards their well-being and enhancing the quality of care provided.

1. Empathy and Compassion:

Empathy and compassion are essential emotional needs of care recipients. Put yourself in their shoes and try to understand their feelings and experiences. Show genuine compassion by acknowledging their challenges, frustrations, and fears. This understanding builds trust and strengthens your relationship with them.

2. Validation and Support:

Care recipients frequently seek validation for their emotions and experiences. Be a supportive presence by actively listening and offering reassurance. Validate their feelings and acknowledge their unique perspective. Ensure they feel heard, understood, and supported in their journey.

3. Respect and Dignity:

Maintaining the care recipient's sense of respect and dignity is crucial for their emotional well-being. Treat them with kindness, patience, and sensitivity. Encourage their independence and involve them in decision-making regarding their care, when possible. Respect their autonomy and preferences, making them feel valued and in control.

4. Communication and Companionship:

Meaningful communication and companionship are vital emotional needs for care recipients. Engage in open and honest conversations, showing your genuine interest in their thoughts and feelings. Create opportunities to spend quality time together, engaging in activities they enjoy. Establishing a strong emotional connection can greatly enhance their sense of well-being.

5. Emotional Stability and Reassurance:

Care recipients may experience emotional instability due to their health condition or the challenges they face. Offer consistent emotional support and reassurance during difficult moments. Be a calming presence, providing stability and helping them navigate their emotions with understanding and patience.

6. Privacy and Personal Boundaries:

Respecting privacy and personal boundaries is crucial for preserving a care recipient's emotional well-being. Allow them to have personal space and time alone as needed. Avoid discussing sensitive topics unless they express a desire to engage in conversations about them. Recognize and honor their need for personal boundaries.

7. Emotional Expression and Outlets:

Encourage care recipients to express their emotions freely and provide them with outlets for emotional release. Encourage journaling, art therapy, or engaging in activities that allow them to express themselves creatively. Foster an open and non-judgmental environment, where they feel safe to express their emotions without fear of criticism.

8. Mental Health Support:

Caregivers should be aware of the potential impact that caregiving can have on a care recipient's mental health. Be vigilant for signs of depression, anxiety, or other mental health concerns. Encourage them to seek professional help if needed and provide resources for counseling or therapy services.

Understanding the emotional needs of care recipients is essential to provide holistic care. By practicing empathy, compassion, and validation, respecting their dignity and autonomy, fostering open communication and companionship, ensuring emotional stability and reassurance, respecting their privacy and personal boundaries, and encouraging emotional expression and mental health support, you create an environment that nurtures their emotional well-being. Remember that each care recipient is unique in their emotional needs, and being attuned to their individuality will help you provide the emotional support they genuinely require.

Caregiving can be emotionally and physically demanding, often leading to stress and burnout. It is crucial for caregivers to prioritize self-care and implement effective strategies to manage stress and prevent burnout. This chapter aims to guide caregivers in recognizing the signs of stress and burnout and providing practical strategies to promote their own well-being.

1. Recognizing the Signs of Stress and Burnout:

Be aware of the signs and symptoms of stress and burnout, which may include feelings of exhaustion, irritability, sleep disturbances, changes in appetite, withdrawal from activities, and a decline in your own physical and mental health. Recognizing these signs early allows you to take proactive steps to address them.

2. Prioritizing Self-Care:

Make self-care a priority in your daily routine. This includes setting aside time for activities that bring you joy and relaxation. Engage in hobbies, exercise regularly, and practice relaxation techniques such as meditation or deep breathing exercises. Prioritize getting adequate sleep and maintaining a healthy diet.

3. Seeking Support:

Don't hesitate to reach out for support when needed. Seek help from friends, family, or support groups specifically designed for caregivers. Sharing your experiences, concerns, and emotions with others who understand your situation can alleviate stress and provide a sense of relief.

4. Setting Realistic Expectations:

Recognize that you cannot do everything and set realistic expectations for yourself. Understand your limitations and establish boundaries to prevent overwhelming yourself. Learn to say no when necessary and delegate tasks to other family members or outside resources when possible.

5. Accepting Help:

Allow others to provide assistance and support. Many people want to help but may not know how. Accept offers of help and be specific about the tasks or responsibilities that others can contribute. Recognize that accepting help benefits both you and your loved one.

6. Time Management and Organization:

Develop effective time management and organizational strategies to help reduce stress. Prioritize tasks and break them down into manageable steps. Create a daily or weekly schedule to provide structure and help prevent overwhelming yourself with too many responsibilities.

7. Engaging in Relaxation Techniques:

Incorporate relaxation techniques into your daily routine to reduce stress. Deep breathing exercises, mindfulness meditation, yoga, or engaging in activities such as listening to calming music or taking a warm bath can help calm your mind and relax your body.

8. Seeking Professional Help:

If stress and burnout become overwhelming, consider seeking professional help from a therapist or counselor. They can provide guidance, support, and coping strategies specifically tailored for caregivers. Therapy can also provide an outlet for processing emotions and finding healthier ways of managing stress.

9. Respite Care:

Utilize respite care services to take periodic breaks from caregiving responsibilities. Respite care allows you to step away temporarily, recharge, and engage in self-care activities. It can involve hiring a professional caregiver or seeking assistance from family members or friends who can provide temporary care for your loved one.

Taking care of your own well-being is essential for being an effective caregiver. By recognizing the signs of stress and burnout, prioritizing self-care, seeking support, setting realistic expectations, accepting help, managing time effectively, engaging in relaxation techniques, considering professional help, and utilizing respite care, you can manage caregiver stress and prevent burnout. Remember that caring for yourself is not selfish; it is necessary to ensure you can provide the best care for your loved one.

Building a Support Network as a Caregiver

Being a caregiver can be a challenging and isolating role. The responsibilities can often feel overwhelming, both physically and emotionally. However, building a support network can provide you with the strength, resources, and encouragement needed to navigate this journey. In this chapter, we will explore strategies to help you build a robust support system that will support your role as a caregiver.

Identifying Your Needs and Resources:

Before reaching out for support, it's important to assess your specific needs as a caregiver. Take some time to reflect on the areas where you require assistance. These may include emotional support, respite care, information about local services, or financial help. Once you have a clear understanding of your needs, you can start exploring the available resources.

1. Family and Friends:

The first step in building your support network is to reach out to your family and friends. Share your caregiving responsibilities with them and explain the specific kind of support you require. You may find that loved ones are more than willing to help once they understand your needs. They can assist with daily tasks, provide emotional support, or even accompany you on medical appointments. Be open and honest about your needs, as people often want to help but may not know how.

2. Caregiver Support Groups:

Connecting with other caregivers who are facing similar challenges can be an invaluable source of support. Look for local support groups, either in-person or online, where you can share your experiences and gain insights from others who have been through similar situations. These groups offer a safe and non-judgmental space to discuss your struggles and learn coping strategies. Professional organizations or local hospitals often organize caregiver support groups.

3. Community Resources:

Explore community programs and services designed to support caregivers. Local organizations such as the Alzheimer's Association, the American Cancer Society, or senior citizen centers may offer information, educational programs, and support services. Contact your local government office or social services department to inquire about available resources in your area. These resources can provide information on specific diseases or conditions, respite care, financial assistance, and support services.

4. Seek Professional Help:

Caregiving can take a toll on your mental and emotional well-being. It's crucial to prioritize your own mental health. Consider reaching out to mental health professionals like therapists or counselors who specialize in caregiver support. They can provide guidance, coping strategies, and help you navigate the challenges of caregiving. Don't hesitate to seek their assistance when needed.

5. Respite Care:

Taking regular breaks is essential to prevent caregiver burnout. Respite care offers temporary relief to caregivers by stepping in and providing care while you take a break. Look for respite programs in your area, such as home health agencies or adult day care centers that offer a few hours or days of respite. Utilizing respite care allows you to recharge and attend to your own personal needs, ensuring you can continue providing quality care.

6. Self-Care:

Maintaining self-care is vital when building a support network. Prioritize your own physical and mental well-being. Practice self-care activities that help reduce stress, such as exercise, meditation, engaging in hobbies, or spending time with friends and loved ones. Taking care of yourself will positively impact your ability to care for others.

Building a support network as a caregiver is essential to sustain your well-being and effectively fulfill your caregiving responsibilities. Identifying your needs, reaching out to family and friends, joining support groups, utilizing community resources, seeking professional help, and practicing self-care are crucial steps in building a strong support system. Remember that asking for help is not a sign of weakness but a necessary step towards ensuring you can provide the best care possible. By building a support network, you will find the strength and encouragement needed to navigate the challenges of caregiving.

Chapter 6

Daily Caregiving Skills

Daily caregiving involves a wide range of essential skills that are necessary to provide optimal care and support for individuals who need assistance with their activities of daily living (ADLs). These skills are crucial in maintaining the health, safety, and well-being of the care recipient. In this chapter, we will explore some key daily caregiving skills that caregivers should develop and practice to enhance the quality of care they provide.

1. Personal Hygiene Assistance:

Assisting with personal hygiene is an essential daily caregiving skill. This includes helping the care recipient with tasks such as bathing, dressing, grooming, and oral care. Caregivers should be knowledgeable about the appropriate techniques and products to use, and be able to respect the care recipient's preferences and independence while providing assistance. Communication and sensitivity are paramount in ensuring that the care recipient feels comfortable and supported during these personal tasks.

2. Mobility and Transfers:

Providing assistance with mobility and transfers is crucial for individuals with limited or compromised mobility. Caregivers should learn proper techniques for assisting with walking, transferring to and from beds or chairs, and using mobility aids such as wheelchairs or walkers. Understanding body mechanics, using proper equipment, and maintaining a safe environment are crucial for preventing injuries to both the caregiver and care recipient.

3. Medication Management:

Many individuals under caregiving require assistance with medication management. Caregivers should develop skills in properly administering medications, understanding dosage instructions, and recognizing potential side effects or adverse reactions. It is essential to maintain accurate documentation, observe schedules, and facilitate effective communication with healthcare professionals. Caregivers should also be vigilant about medication storage, ensuring prescriptions are filled on time, and following medication safety guidelines.

4. Meal Planning and Preparation:

Promoting healthy nutrition and adequate hydration is part of a caregiver's responsibility. Caregivers should have a good understanding of dietary requirements and restrictions, and be able to plan and prepare meals accordingly. This includes meal planning, grocery shopping, meal preparation techniques, and adapting meals to any specific dietary needs or preferences. Being aware of food safety practices is crucial to avoid foodborne illnesses and maintain a healthy environment in the care recipient's home.

5. Incontinence Care:

Providing assistance with incontinence care is a common daily caregiving responsibility. Caregivers should understand the different types of incontinence and be knowledgeable about the appropriate techniques and products for managing it. Maintaining dignity, respecting privacy, and adhering to infection control practices are essential while providing incontinence care.

6. Cognitive Stimulation and Mental Health Support:

Daily caregiving involves providing emotional support and cognitive stimulation to care recipients, especially those with cognitive impairments. Caregivers should develop skills in engaging individuals with meaningful activities, supporting memory retention techniques, and fostering a positive and stimulating environment. It is crucial to be patient, compassionate, and observant of changes in behavior or mood that may indicate mental health concerns.

Mastering daily caregiving skills enhances the quality of care provided to individuals who require assistance with their activities of daily living. By developing expertise in personal hygiene assistance, mobility and transfers, medication management, meal planning, incontinence care, and cognitive stimulation, caregivers can ensure the safety, well-being, and overall quality of life for care recipients. Continued learning, effective communication, and empathy are fundamental aspects of daily caregiving.

Basics of Personal Care Assistance

Personal care assistance is a fundamental aspect of caregiving that involves providing support and assistance to individuals who have difficulty performing their activities of daily living (ADLs) independently. This chapter will focus on the basics of personal care assistance, including key skills and techniques that caregivers should possess to provide effective and compassionate care.

1. Understanding Activities of Daily Living (ADLs):

To provide adequate personal care assistance, caregivers must have a clear understanding of the activities of daily living. ADLs typically include tasks such as bathing, dressing, grooming, toileting, eating, and transferring. Caregivers should recognize the importance of maintaining dignity, promoting independence, and respecting the preferences and individual needs of the care recipient during the provision of personal care.

2. Safe and Effective Bathing:

Bathing is a crucial aspect of personal care assistance. Caregivers should ensure the safety and comfort of the care recipient during bathing. This may involve helping the individual get in and out of the bath or shower safely, providing appropriate bathing aids such as shower chairs or handrails, and using techniques to minimize the risk of accidents or falls. Caregivers should also be conscious of privacy and maintain a respectful and dignified environment during bathing.

3. Dressing and Grooming Support:

Assisting with dressing and grooming requires caregivers to be mindful of the care recipient's preferences and abilities. Caregivers should communicate effectively to understand the individual's style, comfort, and any physical limitations they may have. Skills in selecting appropriate clothing, helping with dressing, and assisting with grooming tasks like hair care, shaving, and oral hygiene are essential for promoting personal hygiene and maintaining self-esteem.

4. Toileting Assistance:

Providing toileting assistance can be sensitive and challenging for both caregivers and care recipients. Caregivers should prioritize the individual's privacy, dignity, and independence whenever possible. This may involve assisting with transferring to and from the toilet, using appropriate toileting aids such as commode chairs or grab bars, and handling incontinence issues with empathy and discretion. Clear and open communication is crucial in ensuring the care recipient's comfort and overall well-being.

5. Supportive Eating and Drinking:

Assisting individuals with eating and drinking involves more than just providing meals. Caregivers should be aware of any dietary restrictions or modifications required and ensure that meals are nutritionally balanced and appealing. They should also be proficient in feeding techniques, assisting with proper positioning, and taking precautions to prevent choking or aspiration. Promoting hydration and mindful eating practices is crucial for maintaining the individual's overall health and well-being.

6. Transferring and Mobility Aid Techniques:

Many individuals requiring personal care assistance may have limited mobility or require the use of mobility aids. Caregivers should be knowledgeable in safe transferring techniques, using equipment such as transfer belts or slide boards as necessary. Understanding body mechanics and proper handling practices help prevent injuries to both the caregiver and care recipient. Additionally, assisting with walking, moving within the home, or using assistive devices like canes or walkers may be necessary.

The basics of personal care assistance involve understanding the activities of daily living and providing support and assistance to individuals who need help with their personal care routines. By mastering skills in safe and effective bathing, dressing and grooming support, toileting assistance, supportive eating and drinking, and transferring and mobility aid techniques, caregivers can enhance the care recipient's physical and emotional well-being. Empathy, patience, and respect are integral to providing dignified and compassionate personal care assistance.

Administering Medications and Medical Tasks

Administering medications and performing medical tasks are vital responsibilities of caregivers, especially when caring for individuals with chronic health conditions or those who require specialized medical interventions. This chapter will provide an overview of the essential skills and considerations caregivers should have when managing medications and performing medical tasks to ensure the safety and well-being of the care recipient.

1. Understanding Medications:

One of the crucial aspects of administering medications is the caregiver's understanding of the medications prescribed to the care recipient. Caregivers should familiarize themselves with the purpose, dosage, potential side effects, and any contraindications or interactions. Reading and comprehending medication labels, instructions, and warning signs are essential to ensure accurate administration.

2. Medication Management and Organization:

Maintaining accurate and organized medication records is critical for effective medication management. Caregivers should be skilled in keeping track of medication schedules, ensuring timely refills, and maintaining clear communication with healthcare professionals regarding any changes in medications. Developing a system for organizing and storing medications safely, such as using pill organizers or labeled medication containers, helps prevent errors and improve medication adherence.

3. Safe Medication Administration:

To safely administer medications, caregivers should follow healthcare providers' instructions and adhere to established protocols. This includes verifying the correct medication, dosage, and route of administration before giving any medication. Caregivers must also be knowledgeable about different medication administration techniques, such as oral, topical, subcutaneous, or intramuscular routes, and be trained in using medical devices like syringes or inhalers.

4. Observing and Documenting Medication Effects:

Caregivers play a crucial role in observing and documenting the effects of medications on the care recipient's health and well-being. This involves monitoring for any adverse reactions or side effects, changes in vital signs, or improvements in symptoms. Careful documentation helps facilitate effective communication with healthcare professionals and ensures that medication adjustments can be made if necessary.

5. Basic First Aid and Emergency Response:

Having basic first aid skills is essential for caregivers, as they may need to handle minor injuries or respond to medical emergencies. Caregivers should be trained in CPR (cardiopulmonary resuscitation) and basic life support techniques to provide immediate assistance in critical situations. Being prepared with a fully stocked first aid kit, knowing emergency contact numbers, and having a clear plan in place are vital for managing emergencies effectively.

6. Specialized Medical Tasks:

Some care recipients may require specialized medical tasks, such as wound care, administering injections, managing medical equipment, or monitoring vital signs. Caregivers should receive proper training, either from healthcare professionals or specialized training programs, to handle such tasks safely and effectively. Following established protocols, maintaining cleanliness and infection control measures, and being proactive in seeking guidance or clarification when needed are crucial for performing these tasks accurately.

Administering medications and performing medical tasks are integral parts of caregiving. By understanding medications, organizing and managing them effectively, safely administering medications, monitoring effects, and being prepared for emergencies, caregivers can ensure the care recipient's medication adherence, safety, and overall well-being. Seeking proper training, staying updated on medical information, and maintaining open communication with healthcare professionals are essential to provide competent and quality care in these areas.

Safety Measures and Fall Prevention

Safety measures and fall prevention are of utmost importance in caregiving, as falls pose a significant risk to the well-being and independence of individuals who require assistance. This chapter will focus on understanding the importance of safety measures, identifying potential hazards, and implementing strategies to prevent falls and promote a safe environment for the care recipient.

1. Importance of Safety Awareness:

Creating a culture of safety awareness is crucial for caregivers. It involves being vigilant and proactive in identifying potential hazards and taking necessary precautions to minimize risks. Caregivers should recognize the importance of their role in preventing accidents, maintaining a safe home environment, and promoting the care recipient's confidence and independence.

2. Home Safety Assessment:

Conducting a comprehensive home safety assessment is an essential step in preventing falls. Caregivers should pay attention to potential hazards such as inadequate lighting, slippery floors, loose carpets, cluttered pathways, and uneven surfaces. They should identify and rectify these hazards by installing grab bars, securing rugs, removing obstacles, improving lighting, and ensuring a clear and accessible home layout.

3. Fall Prevention Strategies:

Implementing strategies to prevent falls is key in ensuring the safety of the care recipient. Caregivers should encourage the use of assistive devices such as walkers or canes, and ensure that they are properly fitted and maintained. Clear pathways, removing tripping hazards, and using non-slip mats and rugs can significantly reduce the risk of falls. Additionally, helping the care recipient with proper footwear and encouraging regular exercise for strength and balance can further enhance fall prevention efforts.

4. Bathroom Safety:

The bathroom is an area prone to falls and accidents. Caregivers should install grab bars near the toilet, bath, and shower areas to provide stability and support. Non-slip mats or adhesive strips can be placed in the shower or bathtub to improve traction. Adequate lighting and easy-to-reach essentials, such as towels or soap, should also be ensured. Regular cleaning to prevent slippery surfaces is important as well.

5. Adequate Lighting:

Proper lighting is essential for creating a safe and visible environment for the care recipient. Caregivers should ensure that there is sufficient lighting throughout the home, especially in stairways, hallways, and frequently used areas. Nightlights or motion sensor lights can be placed to help individuals navigate safely, especially during nighttime trips to the bathroom.

6. Education and Communication:

Educating the care recipient about fall prevention measures and actively engaging them in the process is crucial. Caregivers should communicate the importance of safety measures and involve the care recipient in identifying potential hazards and taking appropriate preventive measures. Open communication helps in addressing concerns, adapting the environment to individual needs, and reinforcing safe practices.

7. Regular Review and Adaptation:

Safety measures and fall prevention strategies should be regularly reviewed and adapted to meet the changing needs of the care recipient. Caregivers should assess the effectiveness of implemented measures, address new or emerging hazards, and modify safety plans as required. Regular communication with healthcare professionals and seeking their expertise can also provide valuable insights and recommendations.

Prioritizing safety measures and fall prevention is essential in providing a secure and supportive environment for the care recipient. By conducting home safety assessments, implementing fall prevention strategies, ensuring bathroom safety, promoting adequate lighting, actively involving the care recipient, and regularly reviewing and adapting safety measures, caregivers can significantly reduce the risk of falls and enhance the overall well-being of the individual under their care. Continued vigilance and communication with healthcare professionals play a vital role in maintaining a safe and secure caregiving environment.

Chapter 7:

Dealing with common health issues

]

As a caregiver, it is crucial to be prepared and knowledgeable about common health issues that may arise when caring for an individual. This chapter will explore some of the most frequent health issues caregivers may encounter and provide essential information on how to manage and support the care recipient effectively.

1. Respiratory Issues:

Respiratory issues, such as coughing, shortness of breath, or respiratory infections, are common health concerns. Caregivers should encourage good respiratory hygiene, which includes covering the mouth and nose when coughing or sneezing and proper disposal of tissues. Maintaining a clean and dust-free environment, adequate ventilation, and proper hydration can also help support respiratory health. If necessary, caregivers should seek medical attention promptly and follow prescribed treatments or medications.

2. Skin Care:

Proper skin care is essential to prevent skin breakdown, pressure ulcers, and infections. Caregivers should ensure the care recipient's skin is clean, dry, and moisturized. Regularly inspecting the skin for redness, irritation, or any changes is important. Following appropriate hygiene practices, using mild cleansers, and implementing a turning and repositioning schedule can minimize the risk of pressure sores. Seeking medical advice for any concerning skin conditions or changes is recommended.

3. Digestive Issues:

Digestive issues, such as constipation, diarrhea, or indigestion, can impact the care recipient's overall well-being. Caregivers should encourage a balanced diet rich in fiber and fluids to promote regular bowel movements. Maintaining proper hydration, encouraging physical activity, and assisting with toileting as needed can all support digestive health. In case of persistent or severe symptoms, caregivers should consult healthcare professionals for further guidance.

4. Urinary Tract Infections (UTIs):

UTIs are common infections among individuals requiring caregiving. Caregivers should ensure the care recipient maintains good personal hygiene, including regular and thorough cleaning of the genital area. Encouraging adequate fluid intake and frequent bathroom breaks are also crucial. Recognizing the signs of UTIs, such as pain or discomfort during urination, cloudy urine, or strong-smelling urine, is important. If UTI symptoms arise, caregivers should seek medical attention promptly for proper diagnosis and treatment.

5. Musculoskeletal Issues:

Musculoskeletal issues, including arthritis, muscle strains, or joint pain, can cause discomfort and limit mobility. Caregivers should encourage regular physical activity and gentle exercises, such as stretching or range-of-motion exercises, to help maintain joint flexibility and muscle strength. Providing assistance with activities that may cause strain or injury and using assistive devices, such as canes or walkers, can support proper body mechanics and reduce the risk of musculoskeletal issues. Seeking medical guidance for pain management and appropriate treatment options is important as well.

6. Mental Health Concerns:

Caregivers should be vigilant about mental health concerns, as they can significantly impact the well-being of the care recipient. Recognizing signs of depression, anxiety, or cognitive decline is crucial. Engaging in meaningful activities, maintaining social connections, and providing emotional support and reassurance are essential. Encouraging the care recipient to communicate their feelings and ensuring access to mental health resources, such as therapy or counseling, when necessary, is vital. Collaboration with healthcare professionals is important to address any mental health issues effectively.

7. Medication Side Effects:

Medication side effects can occur, and caregivers should be observant and knowledgeable about potential adverse reactions. Caregivers should be familiar with the prescribed medications, read and understand the accompanying information, and follow healthcare professionals' instructions. Observing and reporting any unusual or concerning symptoms promptly to the healthcare team is crucial. Regular communication with healthcare professionals ensures proper monitoring and adjustment of medications if needed.

Dealing with common health issues is an integral part of caregiving. By being prepared, knowledgeable, and proactive, caregivers can effectively manage and support individuals with respiratory issues, skin care needs, digestive issues, UTIs, musculoskeletal concerns, mental health challenges, and potential medication side effects. Regular communication and collaboration with healthcare professionals, along with maintaining a supportive and caring approach, are key in ensuring the care recipient's overall well-being and quality of life.

Recognizing Common Health Issues

One of the crucial aspects of maintaining good health is the ability to recognize common health issues. Often, certain symptoms or warning signs indicate underlying conditions that, if detected early, can be managed or treated more effectively. In this chapter, we will explore several health issues that are frequently encountered and provide guidance on how to recognize them accurately.

Section 1: Respiratory Issues

1. Asthma: Recognizing symptoms such as frequent coughing, wheezing, shortness of breath, and chest tightness can help identify asthma. Its severity can vary, so it is crucial to consult a healthcare professional for proper diagnosis and management.

2. Chronic Obstructive Pulmonary Disease (COPD): COPD primarily affects smokers or those exposed to certain chemicals. Symptoms include persistent coughing, wheezing, shortness of breath, and frequent respiratory infections. Recognizing these symptoms is essential for early intervention, as COPD can be better managed in its initial stages.

Section 2: Cardiovascular Issues

1. High Blood Pressure (Hypertension): Hypertension is often referred to as the "silent killer" due to its lack of noticeable symptoms. Regular monitoring of blood pressure is crucial, as persistent high blood pressure can lead to heart disease or stroke.

2. Coronary Artery Disease (CAD): Recognizing symptoms like chest pain or discomfort (angina), shortness of breath, and fatigue, particularly during physical exertion, can help identify CAD. Prompt medical intervention can prevent further complications such as heart attack or heart failure.

Section 3: Gastrointestinal Issues

1. Gastroesophageal Reflux Disease (GERD): GERD causes frequent heartburn or acid reflux, often accompanied by regurgitation of stomach acid. These symptoms, if recurring, can indicate GERD, which may require lifestyle modifications, medication, or further investigation by a healthcare professional.

2. Irritable Bowel Syndrome (IBS): Frequently experiencing abdominal pain, bloating, changes in bowel movements, and mucus in the stool could indicate IBS. Identifying and managing triggers, stress reduction, and dietary changes can significantly improve quality of life for those with IBS.

Section 4: Mental Health Issues

1. Depression: Recognizing persistent feelings of sadness, hopelessness, loss of interest in previously enjoyed activities, changes in appetite, sleep disturbances, and thoughts of self-harm is crucial to identifying and seeking help for depression.

2. Anxiety Disorders: Symptoms such as excessive worry, restlessness, irritability, difficulty concentrating, and physical symptoms like rapid heartbeat or shortness of breath can suggest an anxiety disorder. Early intervention and appropriate treatment are essential to managing anxiety effectively.

Recognizing common health issues is vital for early intervention and effective management. Being aware of the symptoms associated with various conditions can empower individuals to seek appropriate medical help and make necessary lifestyle changes. Regular check-ups, self-awareness, and understanding of these common health issues lay a foundation for maintaining optimal health and well-being. Always consult with a healthcare professional for accurate diagnosis and personalized guidance.

Living with a chronic illness or disability can present unique challenges that require careful management. In this chapter, we will explore strategies and resources to help individuals effectively cope with chronic illnesses and disabilities. By implementing proactive measures and seeking appropriate support, individuals can lead fulfilling lives despite these conditions.

Section 1: Developing a Personalized Care Plan

1. Consultation with Healthcare Professionals: Establishing an ongoing relationship with healthcare providers is crucial for managing chronic illnesses and disabilities. Regular check-ups, medication management, and guidance on lifestyle modifications play a vital role in maintaining overall well-being.

2. Understanding and Monitoring Symptoms: Being knowledgeable about one's condition enables better symptom tracking and identification. By keeping a symptom diary or using technology to monitor health metrics, individuals can communicate effectively with healthcare professionals and make informed decisions regarding their care.

Section 2: Lifestyle Modification and Self-Care

1. Establishing Healthy Habits: Adopting a balanced diet, engaging in regular exercise suitable for individual abilities, managing stress, and getting quality sleep are fundamental for managing chronic illnesses and disabilities. Consulting with healthcare professionals and, if possible, working with a registered dietitian or physical therapist can assist in developing an appropriate lifestyle plan.

2. Medication Adherence: Following prescribed medication regimens is crucial to maintain stability and manage symptoms effectively. Utilizing medication organizers, setting reminders, and regularly communicating with healthcare providers about any concerns or side effects can aid in optimal medication management.

Section 3: Emotional Well-being and Support

1. Seeking Emotional Support: Living with chronic illnesses or disabilities may give rise to various emotional challenges. Connecting with support groups, therapy, or counseling can

provide a safe space to discuss feelings, learn coping mechanisms, and receive guidance on managing emotional well-being.

2. Self-Care and Stress Management: Engaging in activities that bring joy, practicing relaxation techniques like deep breathing or mindfulness, seeking hobbies, and setting realistic goals can contribute to better emotional well-being and stress reduction.

Section 4: Utilizing Available Resources

1. Assistive Devices and Accessibility: Depending on the specific chronic illness or disability, utilizing assistive devices such as wheelchairs, hearing aids, or mobility aids can enhance independence and quality of life. Seeking information regarding accessibility services, home modifications, or workplace accommodations can also provide additional support.

2. Government and Community Programs: Investigating available government assistance programs, disability services, and resources such as vocational rehabilitation or support networks can be invaluable in managing chronic illnesses and disabilities. Local community organizations and online communities can provide connections and support from others in similar situations.

While living with chronic illnesses and disabilities presents unique challenges, implementing proactive measures and seeking appropriate support can significantly improve overall well-being. Developing a personalized care plan, making lifestyle modifications, prioritizing emotional well-being, and utilizing available resources empower individuals to manage their conditions effectively and lead fulfilling lives. Remember, individual experiences may vary, and it is important to consult healthcare professionals and specialists for personalized guidance in managing specific chronic illnesses and disabilities.

Communicating with Healthcare Professionals Effectively in Caregiving

When caring for a loved one, effective communication with healthcare professionals becomes even more crucial. As a caregiver, you play a vital role in ensuring that your loved one receives the best possible care. In this chapter, we will explore strategies and techniques to help caregivers communicate effectively with healthcare professionals.

Section 1: Establishing a Partnership

1. Introduce Yourself: When meeting healthcare professionals, introduce yourself as the caregiver and provide relevant information about your role in your loved one's care. This helps establish open lines of communication from the beginning.

2. Build Rapport: Foster a respectful and collaborative relationship with healthcare professionals. Establishing trust and clear communication from the start will facilitate a more effective caregiving experience.

Section 2: Sharing Information

1. Maintain Updated Records: Keep a comprehensive record of your loved one's medical history, including diagnoses, medications, allergies, and past treatments. This information will help healthcare professionals understand your loved one's health status accurately.

2. Communicate Changes: Inform healthcare professionals about any changes in symptoms, behaviors, or conditions your loved one experiences. Sharing these observations will assist in proper diagnosis and treatment planning.

Section 3: Preparation for Appointments

1. Prepare Questions: Make a list of questions or concerns you have before each appointment. This ensures that all important matters are addressed and prevents forgetting any relevant information.

2. Bring Necessary Information: Bring all relevant documents, such as medical records, test results, and a list of medications, to appointments. This provides healthcare professionals with a complete picture of your loved one's health.

Section 4: Effective Communication during Appointments

1. Be Clear and Concise: Clearly articulate your concerns or questions during appointments. Avoid going off-topic and provide concise information to help healthcare professionals understand your needs.

2. Active Listening: Pay close attention to what healthcare professionals say during appointments. Take notes if necessary, and ask for clarification if something is unclear. This will ensure that you fully understand the advice or treatment plan for your loved one.

Section 5: Advocating for Your Loved One

1. Voice Concerns: If you have concerns or doubts about a diagnosis, treatment plan, or medication, communicate them respectfully with healthcare professionals. Your advocacy is essential in ensuring your loved one receives appropriate care.

2. Seek Information: Request explanations about treatment options, potential side effects, or risks involved. Understanding the available options empowers you to make informed decisions for your loved one's health.

Section 6: Maintaining Communication Channels

1. Follow-up Communication: After appointments or hospital visits, provide updates to healthcare professionals if necessary. This ensures continuity of care and supports their decision-making process.

2. Utilize Technology and Telehealth: Leverage technology, such as online portals or telehealth platforms, to communicate with healthcare professionals conveniently. These tools can facilitate communication, reduce travel time, and make healthcare more accessible.

Effective communication with healthcare professionals is vital for caregivers to ensure excellent care for their loved ones. By establishing a partnership, sharing comprehensive information, preparing for appointments, practicing active listening, advocating when necessary, and utilizing available communication channels, caregivers can navigate the healthcare system more effectively. Remember, open and respectful communication benefits both your loved one and the healthcare professionals involved in their care, creating a collaborative team focused on the well-being of your loved one.

Chapter 8

Caring for Dementia and Alzheimer's Patients

Caring for individuals with dementia or Alzheimer's disease requires unique understanding, compassion, and specialized approaches to provide the best possible care. In this chapter, we will explore strategies, techniques, and resources to help caregivers navigate the challenges associated with caring for loved ones with dementia or Alzheimer's disease.

Section 1: Building a Support System

1. Seek Professional Help: Enlist the support of healthcare professionals experienced in dementia and Alzheimer's care. They can provide valuable guidance, information, and assistance in managing the various aspects of caregiving.

2. Join Support Groups: Connecting with other caregivers facing similar challenges can be immensely helpful. Support groups offer a safe space for sharing experiences, advice, and emotional support.

Section 2: Enhancing Communication

1. Simplify Communication: Use clear, simple language and speak slowly to aid comprehension. Maintain a calm and reassuring tone, and allow sufficient time for the person with dementia or Alzheimer's to process and respond.

2. Non-Verbal Communication: Pay attention to non-verbal cues such as facial expressions and body language. These can provide valuable insights into the individual's emotional state or needs.

Section 3: Creating a Safe and Structured Environment

1. Remove Hazards: Ensure the immediate environment is free from potential dangers. Remove obstacles, secure loose rugs, and install safety measures like grab bars to prevent accidents.

2. Establish Routine: Maintain a structured daily routine, as individuals with dementia or Alzheimer's often find comfort and security in predictable patterns. Consistency in meals, activities, and sleep schedules can reduce agitation and confusion.

Section 4: Managing Challenging Behaviors

1. Remain Calm and Patient: When faced with challenging behaviors, staying calm and patient is essential. Take deep breaths, use a reassuring tone, and try redirecting attention to a different activity or topic.

2. Validate Feelings: Acknowledge and validate the emotions expressed by the individual, even if their statements or beliefs do not align with reality. Avoid arguing or attempting to correct their perception, as it often leads to frustration or agitation.

Section 5: Creating Meaningful Activities

1. Engage in Activities: Encourage participation in activities that provide mental stimulation and promote a sense of purpose. Simple tasks such as arts and crafts, puzzles, gardening, or listening to familiar music can bring joy and maintain cognitive function.

2. Adapt Activities: Modify activities to match the individual's current abilities. Break tasks into smaller, manageable steps, provide visual cues or prompts, and offer assistance as needed while encouraging independence.

Section 6: Self-Care for Caregivers

1. Prioritize Self-Care: Caregivers must prioritize their physical and emotional well-being to provide effective care. Set boundaries, seek respite care when needed, and engage in activities that promote relaxation and rejuvenation.

2. Educate Yourself: Stay informed about the progression of dementia and Alzheimer's disease, available resources, and strategies for managing care. Knowledge empowers caregivers to make informed decisions and provide better support.

Caring for individuals with dementia and Alzheimer's disease can be challenging, but with the right techniques and support, it is possible to provide compassionate, effective care. Building a support system, enhancing communication, creating a safe environment, managing challenging behaviors, engaging in meaningful activities, and practicing self-care are all vital aspects of dementia and Alzheimer's caregiving. Remember, each individual's journey is unique, so adaptability and patience are key throughout the caregiving process.

Understanding Dementia and Its Stages

Dementia is a complex and progressive condition that affects cognitive function and memory. Understanding the stages of dementia is essential for caregivers and family members to provide appropriate support and care. In this chapter, we will explore the different stages of dementia and their associated characteristics.

Section 1: Mild Cognitive Impairment (MCI)

1. Overview: Mild Cognitive Impairment is considered a pre-dementia stage, where individuals may experience subtle changes in memory, thinking, or concentration. However, individuals can still perform daily activities independently.

2. Characteristics:

- Forgetfulness of recent events or details.

- Difficulty finding words or recalling names.

- Challenges with complex tasks or planning.

- No significant impact on overall functioning or independence.

Section 2: Early Stage Dementia

1. Overview: Early stage dementia is characterized by noticeable cognitive decline that impacts daily functioning. Memory loss and difficulty with complex tasks become more apparent during this stage.

2. Characteristics:

  - Difficulty with recall and retaining new information.

  - Challenges with problem-solving and planning.

  - Increased confusion in new or unfamiliar environments.

  - Mood swings, irritability, or apathy.

  - Impaired judgment and decision-making abilities.

Section 3: Moderate Stage Dementia

1. Overview: In the moderate stage of dementia, cognitive decline becomes more pronounced, leading to increased dependence on others for daily tasks. Individuals may experience significant memory loss and exhibit behavioral changes.

2. Characteristics:

  - Greater difficulty with short-term memory and recalling recent events.

  - Confusion about time, place, and people.

  - Challenges with basic tasks like dressing, bathing, or managing finances.

  - Agitation, aggression, or wandering.

  - Difficulty expressing thoughts and needs.

Section 4: Severe Stage Dementia

1. Overview: Severe stage dementia is characterized by a significant decline in cognitive function and extensive reliance on others for care. Individuals in this stage may lose the ability to communicate, recognize loved ones, or perform basic tasks.

2. Characteristics:

  - Profound memory loss, including forgetting personal history.

  - Inability to recognize familiar faces or environments.

  - Difficulty swallowing, leading to weight loss.

- Loss of mobility and muscle control.

- Increased vulnerability to infections and other health complications.

Section 5: Palliative or End-Stage Dementia

1. Overview: Palliative or end-stage dementia typically occurs in the final weeks or months of an individual's life. Physical and cognitive decline is extensive, and they require round-the-clock care.

2. Characteristics:

- Inability to communicate verbally.

- Extreme difficulty with mobility and self-care.

- Limited or no ability to eat, swallow, or control bodily functions.

- General weakness, weight loss, and decreased responsiveness.

- Increased vulnerability to infections and other medical complications.

Understanding the stages of dementia provides caregivers and family members with valuable insights into the progression of the condition. Each stage brings unique challenges, and recognizing the associated characteristics allows for appropriate support and care to be provided. It is important to remember that each person's experience with dementia varies, and the pace of progression may differ. Working with healthcare professionals and support organizations can further enhance the understanding of dementia and enable caregivers to provide optimal care and support throughout the various stages.

Strategies for Communication and Engagement with Dementia Patients and Caregivers

Effective communication and meaningful engagement are essential components of quality care for people with dementia. Dementia not only affects memory and cognitive functions but also impairs the individual's ability to communicate and engage with others. In this chapter, we will explore various strategies that healthcare professionals, caregivers, and family members can employ to enhance communication and engagement with dementia patients. Additionally, we will discuss the importance of engaging with caregivers, providing them with support and resources to improve their own well-being.

1. Enhancing Communication with Dementia Patients:

1.1. Non-verbal Communication: Non-verbal cues such as facial expressions, gestures, and touch play a crucial role in communication with dementia patients. Maintain eye contact, use a warm and friendly tone of voice, and offer reassuring physical contact when appropriate.

1.2. Simplify Language: Use simple, clear, and concise language, avoiding complex sentences and jargon. Break down instructions or questions into individual steps to enhance comprehension.

1.3. Active Listening: Allow ample time for the person with dementia to process and respond to questions or statements. Avoid interrupting or finishing their sentences, as it can be frustrating and discouraging.

1.4. Use Visual Aids: Utilize visual aids, such as photographs, written cues, or symbol charts to supplement verbal communication. This can help individuals with dementia make connections and better understand the intended message.

2. Encouraging Engagement with Dementia Patients:

2.1. Reminiscence Therapy: Engage the individual in reminiscing about past experiences, encouraging positive memories, and providing a sense of validation and purpose. Displaying familiar objects can spark conversations and improve engagement.

2.2. Sensory Stimulation: Incorporate multisensory activities, such as music, aromatherapy, or tactile materials, to engage the senses and evoke positive emotions. Tailor activities to the person's interests, promoting feelings of joy and well-being.

2.3. Validation Therapy: Validate the feelings and experiences expressed by the person with dementia, even if they seem disconnected from reality. Redirecting conversations towards emotions and personal validation can reduce distress and enhance engagement.

2.4. Life Enrichment Programs: Encourage participation in structured programs designed for dementia patients, such as art therapy, gardening, or pet therapy. These activities provide a sense of purpose, promote social interactions, and enhance overall well-being.

3. Supporting Caregivers:

3.1. Education and Training: Provide caregivers with educational resources and training opportunities to better understand dementia and its challenges. Equip them with communication techniques, caregiving strategies, and knowledge of available support services.

3.2. Respite Care: Support caregivers by offering respite care, allowing them to take breaks from their caregiving responsibilities. Respite care can help prevent caregiver burnout, allowing them time for self-care and rejuvenation.

3.3. Support Groups: Facilitate support groups where caregivers can connect with others facing similar challenges. These groups offer a safe space for sharing experiences, gaining emotional support, and learning from one another.

3.4. Access to Resources: Connect caregivers with community resources, such as support hotlines, dementia-friendly organizations, or respite care programs. Providing information about financial aid options and legal guidance can also alleviate caregivers' worries.

Effective communication and engagement strategies are essential when caring for individuals with dementia. By implementing these strategies, healthcare professionals, caregivers, and family members can enhance their interactions, improve the well-being of dementia patients, and provide valuable support to caregivers. By recognizing the importance of engaging with both patients and caregivers, we can aim to create a compassionate and supportive environment for those affected by dementia.

Creating a Dementia-Friendly Environment for Caregiving

Creating a dementia-friendly environment is crucial for providing optimal care and improving the quality of life for individuals living with dementia. As a caregiver, your role involves adapting the physical space and daily routines to meet the unique needs of the person with dementia. In this chapter, we will discuss various strategies and modifications you can employ to create a dementia-friendly environment, ensuring safety, comfort, and meaningful engagement for your loved one.

1. Safety and Accessibility:

1.1. Remove Hazards: Identify and remove potential hazards, such as loose rugs, cluttered walkways, or sharp objects. Ensure that the environment is free from tripping and falling hazards to minimize the risk of accidents.

1.2. Clear Signage: Use clear and easily comprehensible signage throughout the living space. Label doors, cupboards, and drawers with words or pictures to help the person with dementia locate essential items independently.

1.3. Lighting and Contrast: Ensure adequate lighting in all areas to minimize shadows and confusion. Create contrast between objects and their background by using brightly colored or distinctively patterned furniture and decorations, making objects easier to distinguish.

2. Orientation and Familiarity:

2.1. Memory Aids: Place memory aids around the home, such as a whiteboard with important reminders or a calendar to track daily activities. Utilize labeled drawers or bins to help the person locate personal items or clothing.

2.2. Familiar Objects: Surround the person with items they find familiar and meaningful, such as family photographs, favorite books, or cherished memorabilia. These objects can evoke positive memories and provide a sense of comfort and familiarity.

2.3. Visual Cues: Use visual cues to guide the person through the daily routine. For example, hang a picture of a toothbrush near the bathroom to prompt proper hygiene habits. Visual cues can help maintain independence and reduce confusion.

3. Structured and Engaging Activities:

3.1. Daily Routine: Create a predictable and structured daily routine. Maintaining consistency helps individuals with dementia feel more secure and supported. Establish regular mealtimes, scheduled activities, and designated rest periods to provide a sense of stability.

3.2. Meaningful Activities: Incorporate activities that align with the person's interests and abilities. Engage in hobbies or pastimes they enjoy, such as gardening, crafts, or listening to music. Adjust activities to their current capabilities, promoting a sense of purpose and accomplishment.

3.3. Sensory Stimulation: Integrate sensory activities that engage multiple senses. For example, using scented lotions, playing soothing music, or arranging objects with different textures can evoke positive emotions and promote cognitive stimulation.

4. Emotional Well-being:

4.1. Calming Environment: Create a peaceful and calm environment that supports relaxation. Reduce noise levels, use soothing colors, and provide comfortable seating areas. Utilize nature-themed decorations and natural light to enhance a sense of tranquility.

4.2. Emotional Validation: Demonstrate empathy, patience, and understanding. Validate the person's emotions and experiences, even if their communication is challenging. A compassionate and supportive approach can alleviate anxiety and promote emotional well-being.

Creating a dementia-friendly environment involves adapting the physical space, routines, and activities to meet the unique needs of individuals living with dementia. By incorporating the strategies outlined in this chapter, caregivers can prioritize safety, comfort, and engagement for their loved ones. A dementia-friendly environment helps promote independence, reduces confusion, and enhances the overall well-being and quality of life for individuals living with dementia.

Chapter 9

Respite Care and Self-Care in Caregiving

Caregiving for someone with dementia is a demanding and selfless role that can be physically and emotionally taxing. It is crucial for caregivers to take care of themselves and seek respite from their caregiving responsibilities. In this chapter, we will explore the concept of respite care and the importance of self-care in maintaining the well-being of caregivers. We will discuss various strategies and resources available to support caregivers in their journey.

1. Understanding Respite Care:

1.1. Definition: Respite care refers to a temporary break from caregiving responsibilities, allowing caregivers time to rest, recharge, and attend to their own needs. It can take various forms, such as in-home respite care, adult day programs, or temporary residential care.

1.2. Benefits of Respite Care: Respite care provides much-needed relief to caregivers, preventing burnout and allowing them to maintain their physical and mental health. It offers an opportunity for caregivers to engage in self-care activities, attend personal appointments, or simply have some time for themselves.

2. Identifying Respite Care Options:

2.1. In-Home Respite Care: Professional caregivers come to the caregiver's home to provide care for the individual with dementia while the caregiver takes a break. This type of respite care allows the person with dementia to stay in a familiar environment.

2.2. Adult Day Programs: These programs offer supervised activities, social interaction, and personal care services in a structured setting. Care recipients attend during the day while the caregiver takes a break, knowing their loved one is safe and engaged.

2.3. Temporary Residential Care: Short-term stays in residential care facilities, such as assisted living or memory care communities, provide caregivers with extended breaks, typically ranging from a few days to several weeks.

2.4. Respite Care Grants and Support: Explore financial assistance options and respite care grants available through local government agencies, nonprofit organizations, or insurance providers. These resources can help alleviate the financial burden associated with respite care.

3. Embracing Self-Care:

3.1. Prioritize Personal Health: Take care of physical health by eating nutritious meals, exercising regularly, and getting enough sleep. Attend regular medical check-ups and seek treatment for any health concerns promptly.

3.2. Emotional Well-being: Engage in activities that bring joy and relaxation. Practice stress-management techniques, such as deep breathing exercises, mindfulness, or meditation. Seek emotional support from friends, support groups, or professional counselors.

3.3. Time for Yourself: Establish regular breaks and time off from caregiving duties. Use this time to engage in hobbies, pursue personal interests, or simply enjoy activities that bring you fulfillment and rejuvenation.

3.4. Resilience Building: Develop coping strategies and resilience-building techniques to navigate the challenges of caregiving. This may include setting realistic expectations, setting boundaries, and practicing self-compassion.

4. Seeking Support:

4.1. Support Groups: Join support groups specifically designed for dementia caregivers. These groups provide opportunities to connect with others facing similar challenges, share experiences, and gain valuable emotional support and advice.

4.2. Professional Help: Consult with healthcare professionals, including social workers, geriatric care managers, or therapists specializing in caregiver support. These professionals can offer guidance, resources, and coping strategies tailored to your specific needs.

4.3. Respite Care Services: Research and utilize respite care services in your community. Reach out to local agencies, non-profit organizations, or home care providers to explore respite care options available to you.

Respite care and self-care are fundamental aspects of effective caregiving for individuals with dementia. By recognizing the importance of respite care and prioritizing self-care, caregivers can maintain their own well-being, prevent burnout, and provide higher quality care to their loved ones. Through accessing respite care services and engaging in self-care activities, caregivers can find a balance between their caregiving responsibilities and their personal needs, leading to improved overall health and a more fulfilling caregiving experience.

The Importance of Respite Care for Caregivers

Caregiving for a loved one with dementia is an immensely rewarding, yet challenging, role that often requires extensive physical and emotional efforts. One key aspect of ensuring the well-being of caregivers is the incorporation of respite care. In this chapter, we will delve into the importance of respite care, highlighting its benefits for caregivers and the positive impact it can have on their overall health and ability to provide quality care.

1. Preventing Caregiver Burnout:

1.1. Physical and Emotional Exhaustion: Caregiving can take a toll on the caregiver's physical and emotional well-being. The demands of providing 24/7 care, managing medications, and coping with challenging behaviors can lead to exhaustion, stress, and increased risk of mental health issues such as anxiety and depression.

1.2. Balancing Personal and Caregiving Responsibilities: Caregivers often grapple with juggling their caregiving responsibilities alongside work, parenting, or other personal commitments. This constant juggling can create overwhelm and hinder their ability to effectively care for themselves and their loved one.

1.3. Avoiding Caregiver Burnout: Respite care offers a break from caregiving duties, allowing caregivers time to rest, recharge, and tend to their own physical and emotional needs. This temporary reprieve can help prevent caregiver burnout and restore energy and motivation.

2. Maintaining Physical and Mental Health:

2.1. Rest and Recovery: Chronic lack of sleep and physical strain can compromise the caregiver's immune system and overall health. Regular respite care provides an opportunity to catch up on sleep, address personal health concerns, and engage in rejuvenating activities that promote physical well-being.

2.2. Mental and Emotional Well-being: Caring for someone with dementia can be emotionally draining. Constant worry, feelings of guilt, and witnessing the progression of the disease can lead to anxiety and depression. Respite care allows caregivers to prioritize their emotional well-being by seeking therapy, attending support groups, or engaging in activities that bring them joy and relaxation.

3. Preserving Relationship Dynamics:

3.1. Meaningful Relationships: Maintaining relationships with other family members, friends, and partners is crucial for caregivers' social and emotional support. Respite care provides opportunities for caregivers to nurture these relationships by spending quality time with loved ones, strengthening family bonds, and enjoying activities unrelated to caregiving.

3.2. Reducing Caregiver-Burden Conflict: Without occasional breaks, the caregiver's relationship with the individual they care for may become strained. Fatigue and stress can impact patience and empathy, potentially leading to interpersonal conflicts. Respite care offers much-needed space for caregivers to recharge and return to caregiving responsibilities with renewed patience, compassion, and energy.

4. Enhanced Caregiver Effectiveness:

4.1. Improved Care Quality: Caregivers who access respite care are better equipped to provide quality care to their loved ones. A break from constant caregiving allows caregivers to approach their duties with renewed energy, increased focus, and enhanced problem-solving abilities.

4.2. Professional Caregiver Assistance: Respite care services often involve professionals experienced in dementia care, who can offer specialized knowledge and skills to cater to the unique needs of the individual with dementia. By accessing respite care, caregivers can benefit from these professionals' expertise and expand their knowledge in caregiving techniques.

5. Promoting Personal Identity and Self-Care:

5.1. Personal Fulfillment: Caregiving should not overshadow the caregiver's personal identity and interests. Respite care allows caregivers the space and time to engage in activities they enjoy, pursue hobbies, and fulfill personal goals, thereby promoting a sense of fulfillment and personal growth.

5.2. Self-Care and Well-being: Prioritizing self-care is essential for caregivers to maintain their health, happiness, and ability to provide care. Respite care enables caregivers to engage in self-care practices such as exercise, attending medical appointments, participating in support groups, or simply relaxing and rejuvenating.

Respite care plays a crucial role in supporting and sustaining the well-being of caregivers. By providing temporary relief from caregiving responsibilities, respite care allows caregivers to maintain their own physical and mental health, preserve relationships, enhance their effectiveness as caregivers, and promote personal identity and self-care. Prioritizing respite care not only benefits caregivers but also greatly impacts the quality of care provided to individuals with dementia. By recognizing the importance of respite care, caregivers can ensure longevity and fulfillment in their caregiving journey.

Exploring Respite Care Options as a Caregiver

Being a caregiver can be a rewarding, yet challenging role. It is essential to recognize the importance of taking care of yourself as well. One way to ensure this is by exploring respite care options. Respite care offers temporary relief for primary caregivers, enabling them to take a break, recharge, and focus on their own well-being. In this chapter, we will delve into the various respite care options available and how you can go about exploring and accessing them.

1. Understanding Respite Care:

Respite care refers to a short-term service that provides relief for primary caregivers. It can range from a few hours to several weeks and can be provided in various settings, such as in-home care, adult day centers, or residential facilities. Respite care ensures that caregivers can take time off while ensuring their loved ones receive proper care and support.

2. Types of Respite Care:

a. In-Home Respite Care: In-home respite care involves hiring a professional caregiver who comes to your home and provides care for your loved one. This option allows you to take a break while ensuring your loved one's daily needs are met.

b. Adult Day Care: Adult day centers offer a safe and supportive environment for seniors and individuals with disabilities during the day. Choosing an adult day center allows you to drop off your loved one for a specified amount of time, giving you time and freedom to attend to your own needs.

c. Residential Respite Care: If you need a more extended break or have other commitments, residential respite care may be an option. This entails temporarily placing your loved one in an assisted living facility or nursing home for a specified period.

3. Finding Respite Care Options:

a. Researching Local Resources: Start by researching local resources in your community. Speak to social workers, healthcare professionals, or support groups focused on caregiving. They may provide valuable information on respite care providers or community organizations offering such services.

b. Utilizing Online Resources: Many online platforms and websites provide directories, reviews, and information on respite care services. Explore these resources, read reviews, and compare options to find the most suitable fit for your loved one's needs.

4. Assessing and Selecting Respite Care Providers:

a. Interviewing Potential Providers: Prioritize safety and the level of care offered when selecting a respite care provider. Conduct interviews to get a sense of their qualifications, experience, and suitability for your loved one's specific needs.

b. Checking References and Reviews: Request references from potential providers and speak to other families who have utilized their services. Online reviews and testimonials can also be insightful in gauging the quality of care provided.

c. Facility Visits: If considering residential respite care, visit the facilities personally to observe the environment, cleanliness, and interactions between staff and residents. Trust your instincts and make sure it aligns with your expectations.

5. Funding Respite Care:

a. Insurance Coverage: Check your loved one's health insurance policy for any coverage towards respite care services. Some long-term care insurance policies may cover respite care expenses partially or in full.

b. Government Assistance Programs: Explore government-funded programs that offer financial aid or vouchers specifically for respite care.

c. Non-Profit Organizations and Grants: Research non-profit organizations and foundations that provide grants or funds to assist caregivers with respite care costs. These organizations often aim to improve the quality of life and support for caregivers.

Exploring respite care options can significantly benefit both you as a caregiver and your loved one. Taking the time off to rest, relax, and attend to your own needs is crucial for maintaining your own physical and mental health. By understanding the various types of respite care available, researching local resources, assessing providers, and considering funding options, you can find respite care arrangements that suit your needs and provide a much-needed break. Remember, utilizing respite care services is not a sign of weakness but an acknowledgment of the importance of self-care as a caregiver.

Caregiver Self-Care Practices and Coping Strategies

Being a caregiver can be physically, emotionally, and mentally demanding. To effectively care for others, it is essential to prioritize your own well-being and practice self-care. In this chapter, we will explore various self-care practices and coping strategies that can help caregivers maintain their health, reduce stress, and find balance in their lives.

1. Recognizing the Importance of Self-Care:

Many caregivers feel guilty or selfish when focusing on their own needs. However, self-care is not a luxury but a necessity. Taking care of yourself allows you to provide better care to your loved one. It is essential to understand that self-care is not selfish; it is an act of self-preservation and sustainability.

2. Physical Self-Care:

a. Prioritizing Sleep: Lack of sleep can severely impact a caregiver's physical and mental well-being. Aim for seven to eight hours of quality sleep each night. Establish a bedtime routine, create a comfortable sleep environment, and consider asking for help with nighttime caregiving responsibilities.

b. Healthy Eating: Maintain a balanced diet that includes fruits, vegetables, whole grains, and lean proteins. Eating well provides the necessary energy and nutrients to cope with the demands of caregiving.

c. Regular Exercise: Engage in physical activities that you enjoy and are suitable for your fitness level. Exercise not only benefits your physical health but also releases endorphins, which can improve mood and reduce stress.

3. Emotional and Mental Self-Care:

a. Seek Support: Connect with other caregivers through support groups, online forums, or local community centers. Sharing experiences, challenges, and triumphs with others who understand can be comforting and empowering.

b. Practice Mindfulness and Meditation: Engage in mindfulness exercises, deep breathing techniques, or meditation to calm your mind and reduce stress. These practices can help you stay present and cope with challenging situations effectively.

c. Find Emotional Outlets: Expressing emotions is essential for your well-being. Find healthy outlets such as journaling, art, music, or talking to a trusted friend or therapist. Creating space for emotional release can alleviate stress and provide clarity.

4. Time Management and Boundaries:

a. Set Realistic Expectations: It is crucial to accept that you cannot do everything. Prioritize tasks, delegate when possible, and set realistic expectations for yourself. Accept that perfection is not attainable, and that is okay.

b. Establish Boundaries: Learn to say "no" and set limits on your time and energy. Communicate your boundaries to others, including family members and friends. Setting boundaries allows you to protect your own well-being and prevent burnout.

c. Take Breaks: Schedule regular breaks throughout the day to engage in activities that bring you joy and relaxation. Use these moments as opportunities for self-care and to recharge your batteries.

5. Seeking Professional Help:

a. Therapy or Counseling: If caregiving becomes overwhelming, seek professional help through therapy or counseling. A therapist can provide you with tools and strategies to cope with stress, manage emotions, and navigate the challenges of caregiving.

b. Respite Care: As discussed in the previous chapter, respite care offers temporary relief for caregivers. Utilizing respite care services can give you the much-needed time off to recharge and care for your own needs.

As a caregiver, self-care practices and coping strategies are vital for your well-being and quality of life. Remember, taking care of yourself is not a luxury but a necessity. By implementing physical self-care habits, nurturing your emotional and mental well-being, establishing boundaries, and seeking support, you can cultivate resilience, manage stress, and find balance in your caregiving journey. Prioritizing self-care will not only benefit you but also enhance the quality of care you provide to your loved one.

Chapter 10

Transitioning and Grief in Caregiving

Transitioning is an inevitable part of the caregiving journey, as the health and well-being of your loved one may change over time. As a caregiver, it is essential to navigate these transitions and the accompanying grief effectively. In this chapter, we will explore the challenges of transitioning in caregiving and provide guidance on how to cope with grief during this process.

1. Understanding Transitions in Caregiving:

Caregiving often involves periods of transition as your loved one's health condition evolves. This can include changes in mobility, cognition, independence, or even end-of-life care. Recognizing and accepting these transitions is crucial for both the caregiver and the care recipient.

2. The Grief Process:

a. Anticipatory Grief: While your loved one may still be alive, anticipatory grief refers to the mourning and emotional processing that takes place when caregivers anticipate the loss or changes in their loved one's abilities and health. This grief can occur before or during periods of transition.

b. Ambiguous Loss: Ambiguous loss is a unique type of grief experienced by caregivers, especially when their loved one's condition or prognosis is uncertain. This type of grief can create emotional pain and confusion as caregivers grapple with the loss while still caring for their loved one.

3. Coping with Transitions and Grief:

a. Seek Support: Connect with others who have gone through similar caregiving experiences. Support groups, therapy, or online forums can provide a safe space to share your feelings, fears, and challenges. Being with others who understand can provide validation, empathy, and practical advice.

b. Educate Yourself: Understanding the changes your loved one may be facing can better prepare you for the transition and the subsequent grief. Research their health condition, talk to healthcare professionals, and ask questions. Knowledge can empower you to provide the best possible care and make more informed decisions.

c. Practice Self-Compassion: It is vital to practice self-compassion and acknowledge that it is normal to experience a wide range of emotions during caregiving and grief. Be gentle with yourself, allow yourself to grieve, and give yourself permission to feel and express your emotions openly.

d. Adapt Your Care Routine: As your loved one's condition changes, you may need to adapt your caregiving routine and seek additional resources or assistance. Be open to asking for help and exploring new options, such as respite care or home healthcare services, to provide the best possible care during transitions.

e. Communicate and Plan Ahead: Engage in open, honest, and compassionate communication with your loved one, family members, and healthcare professionals. Discuss wishes, preferences, and goals for both caregiving and end-of-life care. Engaging in these conversations can help alleviate stress and provide a roadmap for decision-making during transitions.

4. Self-Care and Emotional Expression:

a. Allow Yourself to Grieve: Give yourself permission to grieve the loss of your loved one's previous abilities, the future you had envisioned, or even the loss of your own identity as a caregiver. Acknowledge that grief is a natural response to change and loss.

b. Find Emotional Outlets: Expressing your grief through creativity, journaling, or talking to a trusted friend or therapist can provide comfort and emotional release. Find healthy outlets that allow you to process your emotions and receive support.

c. Practice Self-Care: Engage in self-care practices to nurture your physical, emotional, and mental well-being. Prioritize activities that bring you joy, relaxation, and peace, such as exercise, mindfulness, spending time in nature, or pursuing hobbies.

Transitioning and experiencing grief as a caregiver are challenging and deeply personal processes. By understanding the nature of these transitions, seeking support, educating yourself, adapting your care routine, and practicing self-compassion and self-care, you can navigate these challenging periods more effectively. Remember, grieving is a natural part of caregiving, and it is essential to acknowledge your emotions, seek support, and make choices that prioritize your own well-being. Embrace the journey and the lessons it brings, and remember that you are not alone.

Preparing for End-of-Life Decisions in Caregiving

As a caregiver, one of the most important responsibilities you may face is preparing for end-of-life decisions for your loved one. While it can be a challenging and emotional process, proper planning and open communication can ensure that your loved one's wishes are respected and followed. In this chapter, we will explore the steps to prepare for end-of-life decisions and how to navigate this sensitive topic with compassion and respect.

1. Conversations and Advance Directives:

a. Initiate the Conversation: Begin a dialogue with your loved one about end-of-life wishes, including their preferences for medical treatment, palliative care, and the possibility of hospice. Approach the conversation with empathy, sensitivity, and a willingness to listen.

b. Advance Directives: Encourage your loved one to create or update their advance directives, such as a living will and a durable power of attorney for healthcare. These documents outline their wishes for medical treatment and designate a trusted individual to make healthcare decisions on their behalf.

2. Understanding the Medical System:

a. Familiarize Yourself with Medical Terminology: Learn about the common medical terms and procedures related to end-of-life care. This will help you have more informed discussions with healthcare providers and better understand the options available.

b. Consult the Medical Team: Engage in open and honest conversations with your loved one's medical team. Seek clarification and ask questions about their prognosis, potential treatment options, and the possible benefits and risks associated with each option.

3. Hospice and Palliative Care:

a. Explore the Benefits of Hospice: Hospice care focuses on providing comfort, pain management, and emotional support for individuals with terminal illnesses. Learn about the services and benefits hospice can offer, such as pain management, emotional support, and assistance with end-of-life planning.

b. Palliative Care: Palliative care focuses on improving the quality of life for individuals with serious illnesses, regardless of prognosis. It can be provided alongside curative treatment and aims to address physical, emotional, and spiritual needs.

4. Emotional Support and Decision-Making:

a. Involve Family and Loved Ones: Include family members and loved ones in discussions about end-of-life decisions to ensure everyone's voices are heard and respected. Each individual may have unique perspectives and insights that can contribute to the decision-making process.

b. Seek Professional Guidance: Consult with a social worker, counselor, or geriatric care manager specializing in end-of-life care. They can provide guidance, support, and resources to help navigate the decision-making process and ensure your loved one's wishes are honored.

5. Aftercare and Bereavement Support:

a. Aftercare Planning: Be prepared to handle practical matters after your loved one passes, such as contacting funeral homes, notifying family and friends, and managing financial and legal matters.

b. Seek Bereavement Support: Grief is a natural response to loss. Seek support through bereavement counseling, support groups, or therapy. These resources can provide a safe space to navigate the grieving process and find comfort and healing.

Preparing for end-of-life decisions is an emotional and delicate process for caregivers. By initiating honest conversations, understanding advance directives, becoming familiar with end-of-life care options, involving the medical team and loved ones in decision-making, and seeking support and guidance from professionals, you can ensure that your loved one's wishes are respected and followed. Remember, this journey requires compassion, empathy, and open communication. Preparing for end-of-life decisions is a profound act of love and a way to honor the life and legacy of your loved one.

As a caregiver, you understand the joys and challenges that come with the responsibility of caring for a loved one. However, the emotional toll of caregiving can often lead to feelings of grief and loss. This chapter aims to provide strategies and support for coping with the grief and loss experienced throughout your caregiving journey.

1. Acknowledge and Validate your Feelings:

Grief and loss are normal and natural responses to the challenges of caregiving. It is important to acknowledge and validate your feelings without judgment. Allow yourself the space to mourn the changes in your loved one, the lifestyle adjustments, and the potential impact on your own life. Understand that your emotions are valid and deserve acknowledgment.

2. Seek Support:

Caregivers often find solace in seeking support from others who can empathize with their experiences. Joining a support group, whether in-person or online, can provide a sense of community and understanding. Attending counseling sessions or therapy can also be beneficial, as it offers an outlet for expressing emotions and learning coping mechanisms specific to grief and loss.

3. Take Care of Yourself:

Self-care is crucial when coping with grief and loss in caregiving. Prioritize activities that bring you joy and help alleviate stress. Engage in relaxation techniques such as meditation, deep breathing exercises, or yoga. Maintain a healthy lifestyle by getting enough rest, eating nutritious meals, and regular physical exercise. Remember, taking care of yourself is not selfish; it is necessary for your own well-being and ability to provide care.

4. Share Memories and Stories:

Grief can be an opportunity to celebrate the life, memories, and experiences you have shared with your loved one. Take time to reminisce, share stories, or create a scrapbook. These activities can help you honor your loved one's life and find some solace in the memories you hold dear.

5. Embrace Rituals and Symbolism:

Exploring rituals and symbolism can provide comfort during times of grief and loss. Lighting candles, creating altars, or planting a memorial garden can be meaningful ways to remember your loved one. These acts can serve as a continued connection, offering a sense of peace and acceptance as you navigate through your caregiving journey.

6. Seek Professional Help:

If grief becomes overwhelming, and you find it difficult to move forward, it may be essential to seek professional help. Therapists specialized in grief counseling can provide guidance and support tailored to your needs. They can assist in exploring unresolved emotions, facilitating acceptance, and rebuilding your life in the wake of loss.

7. Accept and Adapt to Change:

Caregiving often entails witnessing the decline of your loved one's health and functioning. Acceptance of the changes that occur can be challenging but is vital for your well-being. Allow yourself the space to grieve the loss of your loved one's previous abilities while focusing on adapting to their current needs. Embracing flexibility and seeking assistance when needed will help alleviate some of the emotional burden you may experience.

Conclusion:

Coping with grief and loss in caregiving can be emotionally draining. Remember to be patient with yourself as you navigate these challenging emotions. Seeking support, practicing self-care, and accepting the changes that occur will help you find solace and maintain your well-being throughout your caregiving journey. Remember, you are not alone, and there is support available to help you cope with grief and loss effectively.

Celebrating the Caregiving Journey

Introduction:

While caregiving can present numerous challenges and require significant sacrifices, it's essential to recognize and celebrate the unique journey you are on. This chapter aims to highlight the importance of finding moments of joy, pride, and gratitude throughout your caregiving experience.

1. Recognize Your Impact:

Acknowledge the significant impact you are making in someone's life as a caregiver. Your selflessness, compassion, and dedication are invaluable. Take pride in the role you play in enhancing the quality of your loved one's life and providing them with comfort, support, and love.

2. Embrace Milestones and Achievements:

In the caregiving journey, both you and your loved one are likely to achieve milestones. These could be small victories, such as successfully completing a challenging task, or larger accomplishments, such as recovering from an illness or reaching a new level of independence. Celebrate these milestones together and acknowledge the progress that has been made.

3. Practice Self-Celebration:

Take time to celebrate yourself as a caregiver. Acknowledge your personal growth, resilience, and unwavering dedication. It is easy to overlook your own achievements and focus solely on the needs of your loved one. However, it is important to celebrate the strength and compassion you have shown throughout your caregiving journey.

4. Express Gratitude:

Cultivating a sense of gratitude can bring joy and appreciation into your caregiving experience. Take a few moments each day to reflect on the things you are grateful for within your caregiving journey. It could be the support you receive from others, the moments of connection and love you share with your loved one, or the personal growth you have experienced. Expressing gratitude can shift your perspective and bring a sense of happiness to your caregiving role.

5. Create Meaningful Traditions:

Developing unique traditions and rituals can contribute to a sense of celebration within caregiving. These traditions could be as simple as sharing a favorite meal together each week, taking a regular nature walk, or engaging in an activity you both enjoy. By incorporating meaningful rituals into your caregiving routine, you can build moments of connection and joy.

6. Seek Support and Share Accomplishments:

Engage with other caregivers and support groups to share your caregiving accomplishments. Online forums, local caregiver groups, or social media platforms can be great spaces to connect with others who understand and appreciate the journey you are on. By sharing your achievements and celebrating those of others, you build a sense of camaraderie and mutual support.

7. Practice Self-Care and Recharge:

Taking care of yourself is crucial for maintaining a positive mindset and a sense of celebration. Prioritize self-care activities that bring you joy and rejuvenation. This could include spending time with friends and loved ones, engaging in hobbies or activities you enjoy, or simply taking moments for relaxation and self-reflection. By ensuring your well-being, you are better equipped to appreciate and celebrate your caregiving journey.

Amidst the challenges of caregiving, it is important to remember to celebrate your journey. By recognizing your impact, embracing milestones, practicing self-celebration, expressing gratitude, creating meaningful traditions, seeking support, and prioritizing self-care, you can find joy and fulfillment in your caregiving experience. Take pride in the positive difference you are making in someone's life and the personal growth you are cultivating along the way. Celebrate every step of this unique and important journey.

In conclusion, caregiving is a complex and demanding role that requires patience, compassion, and sacrifice. While it can be challenging and emotionally draining, it also offers numerous rewards and moments of profound connection. The impact that caregivers have on their loved ones' lives is immeasurable, as they provide comfort, support, and love during times of vulnerability. Caregiving offers an opportunity for personal growth, resilience, and a deeper understanding of the human experience. The moments of joy, the milestones achieved, and the relationships forged throughout the caregiving journey are invaluable and transformative. Despite the difficulties, the rewards of caregiving are immeasurable and enrich the lives of both the caregiver and the recipient of care. Embrace the journey, celebrate the difference you are making, and find fulfillment in the privilege of being a caregiver.

To find caregiving resources in your area, it is recommended to use the following methods:

1. Online Search: Conduct an online search using keywords like "caregiving resources in #####" or "caregiver support services in #####." This can provide you with local organizations, support groups, and services specific to your area.

2. Local Senior Centers: Contact local senior centers or adult daycare centers in the ##### zip code. They often have resources and information for caregivers, including support groups, respite care services, and educational programs.

3. Area Agency on Aging: Get in touch with the Area Agency on Aging (AAA) that serves your zip code. AAA provides information, assistance, and resources for older adults and caregivers. They can guide you to local programs and services.

4. Social Services or Department of Health: Reach out to your local social services or department of health offices. They can provide information about caregiver support programs and resources available in your area.

5. Online Caregiver Platforms: Explore online caregiver platforms or directories that connect caregivers with resources and support. Websites like Care.com, Aging Care, or AARP's Caregiving Resource Center may have resources specific to your area.

Remember to personalize your search by specifying the type of assistance you are seeking, such as respite care, support groups, or financial assistance. Additionally, reaching out to healthcare professionals, social workers, or local hospitals may also provide you with valuable information and referrals.

www.ingramcontent.com/pod-product-compliance
Lightning Source LLC
Chambersburg PA
CBHW061008260726
48661CB00005B/2107

9798857750582